Growing Up In Britain:

Ensuring a healthy future for our children

A study of 0–5 year olds

Growing Up In Britain: Ensuring a healthy future for our children
A study of 0–5 year olds

British Medical Association

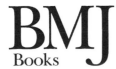

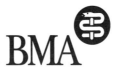

First published in 1999
by BMJ Books, BMA House, Tavistock Square,
London, WC1H 9JP

BMJ Books is an imprint of the BMJ Publishing Group

British Library Cataloguing in Publication Data

A catalogue record for this book is available from the British Library

ISBN 0 7279 1433 2

The photographs on the front cover are reproduced courtesy of Impact Photos.

Typeset by Apek Typesetters, Nailsea, Bristol
Printed and bound by Latimer Trend Ltd, Plymouth

Contents

Editorial Board

Board of Science and Education

This report was prepared under the auspices of the Board of Science and Education of the British Medical Association. The members were:

Working Party

A Working Party with the following membership was set up to advise the Board of Science and Education:

Dr W J Appleyard (Chairman)	Honorary Consultant Paediatrician, Kent and Canterbury Hospitals (NHS) Trust
Professor D J P Barker	Director, MRC Environmental Epidemiology Unit, University of Southampton
Dr R Davies	Consultant Paediatrician
Professor P Graham	Professor of Child Psychiatry
Dr P Leach	Psychologist and writer on child care
Dr C Power	Reader in Epidemiology and Public Health, Institute of Child Health, London
Dr H Roberts	Co-ordinator of Research and Development, Barnardos
Professor J R Sibert	Professor of Community Child Health, University of Wales College of Medicine
Dr J D Watts	General Practitioner, Dundonald, Ayrshire

Acknowledgements

The Association is pleased to acknowledge the help provided by many individuals and organisations in the preparation of this document and we are extremely grateful for the guidance provided by the BMA Craft Committees, and Members of Council. We would also like to thank Professor Stephen Jarvis, Dr Timothy Chambers, Tony Newman, Dr Loretta Light and Dr Jacky Moulton for their help.

Approval for publication as a BMA policy report was recommended by the BMA Council on 9 December 1998.

x

Preface

The purpose of this book is to place the needs of children at the centre of our thinking and prioritise our plans for their future as they grow up in Britain. This aim is not based, as the late James P Grant of UNICEF declared, "on sentimentality or on institutionalised vested interest, but is firmly based on the fact that childhood is a period when the minds and bodies, values and personalities are being formed and during which even temporary deprivation is capable of effecting lifelong damage and distortion of human development – the period of 0–5 years of age is a crucial stage in our early development".

Over the last 100 years many health outcome indicators of children have shown improvement and it is tempting to remain complacent. As a nation we have not made sufficient investment in our children and we have low ratings in comparison to many of our Scandinavian and European colleagues.

The initiative for this study which stimulated debate at the BMA's Annual Representative Meeting, arose from the absence of any specific children's headline targets in the previous government's strategy *The Health of the Nation*. It is interesting to observe that those nations whose mortality statistics for the under fives are among the lowest ten in the world are continually trying to improve their services to children and their families.

This report can be read cover to cover or dipped into as a reference guide to support individual, local and national efforts to put in place practical strategies that will improve our children's health. Sir Donald Court emphasised in his extensive study 20 years ago, that of the legacy of childhood reaching out into adulthood, particularly prominent were the persistent difficulties with disturbed behaviour and emotional control. This topic, together with nutrition, abuse and non-accidental injury, disability and growth, form the five key areas that are highlighted in this volume.

The relative inequalities in the health of our children are increasing. We have examined the evidence of the effectiveness of certain interventions to improve health inequality and we consider the lessons that can be learnt and how they can be applied. A major message is that there is no single answer to one problem, and improvement will require wide-ranging strategies that are developed locally in a multidisciplinary way. Sir Donald

Acheson's detailed report *Inequalities and Health* (1998) stems from the present government's concerns outlined in their document *Our Healthier Nation*. Our book complements the Acheson report and we have developed some of the themes that arose in the section on "Mothers, Children and Families". In particular we have focused on interventions in the under fives where most health gains can be achieved.

I am very grateful to our working party and the interdisciplinary nature of the vigorous discussion that informed this report, and to our referees and many colleagues who have criticised and commented on the text. We view this as the start of an evolving process. The material has had to be selective and condensed and undoubtedly there are gaps that will need to be filled and developed as the dialogue and discussion continue.

Dr James Appleyard
June 1999

Chapter 1 – Introduction

Childhood is a period of rapid and uneven development; physical, psychological, intellectual, emotional and social. Illness, disability and problems of mental health which develop during childhood may remain with an individual throughout life and it is during that childhood that important choices are made and habits adopted which will affect long-term health and well-being. Traumatic effects in childhood such as divorce, unemployment, serious illness, disability or death of a parent or family breakdown may also have profound consequences not only at the time, but in adulthood.

(House of Commons Health Committee, 1997)

The British Medical Association

The British Medical Association (BMA) is the professional organisation representing all doctors in the UK. It was established in 1832 to "promote the medical and allied sciences, and to maintain the honour of the profession". The Board of Science and Education, a standing committee of the Association, supports this aim by acting as an interface between the profession, the government and the public, and by undertaking research studies on behalf of the BMA. Through the publication of policy statements, the Board of Science and Education has led the debate on key public health and professional issues.

The overriding objective of the Board is to contribute to the development of better public health policies that affect the community, the state and the medical profession. In order to do this, investigations are carried out by the Board to examine the impact of various policies and activities on public health. The Board appoints working parties and steering groups, combining medical and other specialist expertise to carry out research on a variety of important issues. The Board has published a large number of reports over recent years reflecting current concerns in public health such as complementary medicine,[1] health inequalities,[2] transport policy and environmental issues,[3,4] the misuse of drugs,[5] domestic violence,[6] and the

1

inequalities of domestic water supply.[7] The Board also has responsibility for educational initiatives. Some reports have been used in medical education programmes, in schools, and higher education. The Board not only develops such educational materials but also has an interest in educational policy.

BMA policy on child health

The BMA has a longstanding interest in issues related to inequalities in society and their impact on health. In 1986 the BMA Annual Representative Meeting (ARM) requested that the Board of Science and Education examine the evidence for a relationship between deprivation and disease. In response to this resolution a working group was established which received evidence from doctors and other experts on many aspects of social disadvantage and its relationship to health. The final report of the working group was published in 1987 entitled *Deprivation and Ill-health.*[8] The report confirmed that social disadvantage makes an important contribution to ill health and examined the possible pathways by which this effect may occur. The BMA continued to monitor the research evidence relating to inequalities in health, and in responding to the 1992 government consultation *The Health of the Nation*,[9] emphasised the importance to health of factors other than those directly related to health care. In 1995 the BMA decided to re-examine the evidence relating to inequalities in health and published an occasional paper of its findings.[2] This paper reported that since 1980 inequalities in income and living standards had increased in the UK. The report of the Commission of Social Justice was considered by the BMA as part of its continuing work on the strategies for tackling inequalities in society and improving public health. The BMA welcomed the report and supported many of the recommendations, viewing these as a means by which inequalities in the UK could be tackled. The BMA's response was published as a report *Strategies for National Renewal: a BMA commentary on the Report of the Commission on Social Justice.*[10]

In 1995 the Annual Representative Meeting of the BMA adopted a resolution requesting that: "the Board of Science and Education prepare a report on 'Growing up in Britain: a healthy future?'" This resolution reflected increasing concern over evidence suggesting that influences early on in life, including during fetal development, affect health in later life. Also of concern were statistics revealing that one in three children lived in poverty.[11] In addition, the resolution clearly related to increasing inequity within Britain in terms of a range of factors including income, health status, and standards of living. A Working Party established to examine these issues concluded that although there would be factors affecting current health and

2

future health throughout childhood and adolescence, it would be of most benefit to focus on the early years of life as they in turn would influence childhood and adolescence.

This current report reflects the conclusions of the earlier BMA report *Inequalities in Health*,[2] which reviewed evidence available since the publication of the Black report,[12] the landmark document that revealed the links between social and economic status and health. Within that BMA report it was suggested that with increasing evidence that health in later life may be dependent on the early years of life, the recommendations of Black with regard to maternity allowances and child health had taken on a particular significance and that the health of young women, pregnant women and young infants should form the focus of attention for policy makers and health professionals.

One of the key themes of the Black report,[12] which has been reiterated by many other researchers since, is that a more holistic approach when treating a presenting problem is required. By defining holistic as taking the whole person into account, these approaches aim for an increase in well-being rather than a reduction in disease and consider social and emotional health as equally important in physical health. As stated by Wilkinson: "the Chancellor has a much greater impact on health than the Secretary of State for Health, a thought that may well not cross the minds of either".[13] This present BMA report examines these broader issues, but with the early years of life as a focus. Although in many areas there is clearly a need for further research, there is sufficient evidence available now to identify a number of the mechanisms by which current and future health relates to factors such as social and economic status. These influences on health can usefully be described as "risk factors" and it is the cumulative effect of risk factors that make poor outcomes more likely. Poverty has been identified as a key risk factor because of the influences it has on many other factors. For example, if a child has a particular physical disability a poorer outcome is more likely when this is combined with poverty. Combining health policy with socio-economic reform is likely to have the greatest effect in terms of reducing the risks to children in lower socio-economic groups, resulting in reduced inequalities in health and improved health for the population as a whole.

The BMA supports the findings of the *Independent Inquiry into Inequalities in Health*,[14] commissioned by the government and chaired by the former Chief Medical Officer, Sir Donald Acheson. The inquiry identified three key areas as being crucial for improvement, recommending that all policies likely to have an impact on health should be evaluated in terms of their impact on health inequalities; a high priority should be given to the health of families with children; and further steps should be taken to reduce income inequalities and improve the living standards of poor households. The BMA welcomes the report's radical agenda to reduce inequalities in health by tackling poverty and in particular the strong emphasis it places on

3

tackling child and maternal poverty. The BMA endorses the conclusion that while there are many interventions which will reduce inequalities between adults, those with the best chance of reducing future inequalities relate to children, to parents and in particular to present and future mothers.[14]

Child health policy in the UK

The Labour government elected in May 1997 has introduced a series of policies and initiatives intended to support families and reduce poverty and social exclusion.[15] In February 1998, they set out their plans to improve the nation's health in the green paper *Our Healthier Nation*.[16] This report appears to herald a total rather than service oriented approach to health, considering the interrelated factors contributing to health inequalities, stating that "connected problems require joined-up solutions". This means tackling inequality which stems from poverty, poor housing, pollution, low educational standards, unemployment, and low pay. Tackling inequalities as a whole is the best means for tackling health inequalities in particular. Child health inequality is considered in the Healthy Schools programme, which includes a commitment to include parenting skills in the school curriculum and encouraging good nutrition in deprived areas by introducing school breakfast clubs. However, it also looks at the wider picture of social and economic inequality, environmental factors and lifestyle decisions (for example smoking and alcohol consumption) which contribute to poor health of family members, including children. Table 1.1 demonstrates the varied major factors affecting health; for many of these factors, the link between poverty and ill health is clear.

The government's recent white paper on tobacco control, *Smoking Kills*, sets out the government's aim to reduce smoking among children from 13%

Table 1.1   Varied major factors affecting health

Fixed	Social and economic	Environment	Lifestyle	Access to services
Genes	Poverty	Air quality	Diet	Education
Sex	Employment	Housing	Physical activity	NHS
Ageing	Social exclusion	Water quality	Smoking	Social Services
		Social environment	Alcohol	Transport
			Sexual behaviour	Leisure
			Drugs	

(Source: Department of Health. *Our Healthier Nation: Green Paper,* CM3852. London: The Stationery Office, 1998. © Crown Copyright material is reproduced with the permission of the Controller of Her Majesty's Stationery Office)

to 9%, and among pregnant women from 23% to 15% by the year 2010. The government has pledged to introduce legislation to ban billboard and press advertising of tobacco at the "earliest practicable opportunity" to dissuade children from smoking.[17]

Parental support schemes

The government plans to fund a National Family and Parenting Institute, set up as an independent charity, and Parentline, a national telephone helpline for parents. These initiatives are intended to support parents and improve parenting skills, though how they will work in practice remains unknown. A number of Early Excellence Centres have been identified, such as the Pen Green Centre described below, and there is a commitment to the development of at least 25 other such centres in areas of socio-economic deprivation.

Pen Green Centre

This centre in Corby, Northamptonshire, provides integrated education, health and social services for more than 300 families each week. In addition to nursery education, there is full time, year-round child care for children aged 18 months to four years. There are also after-school and holiday schemes for older children. A health visitor led child health clinic is held each week, and free pregnancy testing, family planning and legal advice are also available. Parents and other adults are offered a range of literacy, parenting skills and access programmes, and there is a programme of training for workers in the public, private and voluntary sectors. The emphasis on parents' participation and empowerment is particularly strong. The centre is funded by social services and education, with a small contribution from the health authority, and additional charitable and fund-raising income. It is regarded nationally and internationally as a flagship of good practice, though its scale, complexity and cost would make it difficult to replicate in entirety elsewhere.[18]

A budget of £540 million over 3 years has been allocated for a Sure Start programme, targeted at preschool children in areas of high deprivation. It is planned that outreach workers will contact families with children under 3 months old, and work with them to access appropriate local services over the next few years. Child care, primary health care, early education, play, support for parents and other services will be developed in consultation with parents, building on existing services. The Sure Start programme has great potential to support families in need, and tackle health inequalities. One danger is that in the context of so many other initiatives, and with short timescales for planning and implementation, local programmes may be developed with insufficient local consultation, especially with parents, and inadequate training for the workers involved. It is also not clear how the effectiveness of the new programmes will be measured. One encouraging aspect is that Sure Start will be funded via a new Children's Fund, in an administrative structure designed to promote improved communication between government departments.[19] This interdepartmental liaison should help break down some of the divisions which have characteristically hampered early years service provision.

Child care

As part of an approach to welfare reform which encourages movement from benefits and into work, the government has proposed a national child care strategy, with a view to providing more high quality affordable child care for working parents.[20] This includes the provision of free nursery education places for all 4 year olds, with a view to extending this to 3 year olds in the future. This is a welcome development, although it is important to ensure that the education provided is properly tailored to the specific needs of younger children. Other aspects of the child care strategy include: improved training for nursery workers, playgroup leaders, and childminders; standard setting; and coordinated planning at local level led by the local authority but involving other interested parties. Encouraging more uniform, better quality child care is likely to reduce the adverse impact of substandard day care on young children's mental health and cognitive development.

Benefits

The government has introduced several measures designed to reduce child poverty and to increase opportunities for parents of young children to work. It has made a clear commitment to universal child benefit, although the possibility of taxing the benefit of parents in higher income brackets has been raised. The potential benefits from planned rises in child benefit, income support and family credit are offset for some by the loss of lone parent benefit. The introduction of Working Families Tax Credit will help to meet some of the costs of child care for low income families with children. Changes to the way in which Child Support is collected from absent parents will leave parents with care with more income, but may leave non-resident parents on low income worse off.[20] (Barnes M, Child Poverty Action Group, London, personal communication, 1998)

The Welfare to Work policy has less certain benefits in terms of children's mental health. In general, if parents wish to go to work, with good quality child care there should be no adverse effects on the child. But if parents are forced into paid work, this can be a major strain on their capacity to parent adequately.[21] The emphasis of government policy should be more about choice between different options for parents and less about encouraging all parents with very young children to take up paid employment.

Entitlements

In signing the Social Charter, the government has agreed to several European Directives that will benefit working parents with children. For example, one gives both parents the right to 3 months unpaid leave after the birth or adoption of a child (during which time they would receive statutory maternity pay), and the right to take time off for urgent family reasons. Another limits working hours for many people to 48 hours per week and another will help parents who wish to reduce their working hours to do so without losing their employment rights. Although these directives enhance the rights of British parents to spend more time with their young children, many European countries offer much more generous conditions. In France and Finland, for example, mothers with sufficient work histories can stay at home for up to 3 years after the birth of a child or else return to work with subsidised child care. In Austria, mothers can stay at home for 2 years, and in Germany or Sweden for 18 months. Financial support during maternity leave varies from country to country. In Sweden mothers receive full pay for the whole period, and in Finland full pay for the first year.[22]

The importance of having adequate time off work for parents to spend with their children should not be underestimated. Adopting the Social Charter has been seen as a step forward, but to really support families and value parenting, more generous entitlements should be considered.

Delivery of health services

It is difficult to predict how far recent changes to the NHS organisation[23] will impact on the health of young children. Certainly the replacement of annual funding agreements with 3-yearly and sometimes 5-yearly agreements allows for longer term planning and service development. In particular the introduction of Health Action Zones (and similarly Education Action Zones) provides opportunities for innovative multi-agency and public/private sector partnerships in areas of high deprivation, which in principle could enhance the well-being of families with young children.

International child health policy

United Nations Convention on the Rights of the Child, 1991

The Convention was drawn up as an international agreement to protect children's rights.[24] As children have neither a vote nor a public voice, they are more likely than adults to have their rights forgotten or ignored. The UK government in agreeing to be bound by the Convention has to ensure that legislation, and the way in which children are treated in the UK, meets the standards of the Convention. The Convention states that children have three main rights which must be considered whenever any decision is being made about them, or any action is being taken which affects them:

- Non-discrimination: the convention applies to all children equally regardless of race, sex, religion, language, disability, opinion, or family background.
- Best interests: when decisions are made regarding children the best interests of the child must be paramount.
- The child's view: children must be listened to, they have the right to say what they think about any matter that affects them.

Other rights laid down in the Convention relate to civil and political rights, and economic, social, cultural and protective rights. In terms of children's health and well-being the following rights are of importance:

- protection from violence and harmful treatment;
- right to life;
- right to an adequate standard of living;
- right to proper day to day care which encompasses children's rights in terms of separation from parents;
- right to be as healthy as possible;
- right to a healthy environment;
- right to education;
- protection from exploitation.

The UN Convention on the Rights of the Child and the UK government's commitment to the Convention provide a useful framework by which to assess policies in relation to children to ensure that their rights are not overlooked.

WMA Declaration of Ottawa

The World Medical Association (WMA) *Declaration of Ottawa* on the right of the child to health care issued in October 1998 set out several general principles to ensure the health of the child and forms an international bench-mark against which children's services worldwide can be compared.[25] A key principle states that there should be no discrimination in the provision of medical assistance and health care from considerations of age, gender, disease or disability, creed, ethnic origin, nationality, political affiliation, race, sexual orientation, or the social standing of the child or his/her parents or guardians.

The WMA statement on the *International Code of Breastfeeding* also says that parents and children should have access to, and full support in the application of basic knowledge of child health and nutrition, including the advantages of breastfeeding, and the prevention of accidents.

WHO/UNICEF International Code of Marketing of Breastmilk Substitutes

The WHO/UNICEF *International Code of Marketing of Breastmilk Substitutes* was adopted by a resolution of the World Health Assembly in 1981. The International Code bans all promotion of bottle feeding and sets out requirements for labelling and information on infant feeding. Any activity which undermines breastfeeding also violates the aim and spirit of the Code. The Code and its subsequent World Health Assembly Resolutions are intended as a minimum requirement in all countries. The Code believes that the governments of Member States have important responsibilities and a prime role to play in the protection and promotion of breastfeeding as a means of improving infant and young child health. In particular, the Code states that Member States should ensure that appropriate measures are taken including health information and education in the context of primary health care to encourage breastfeeding; and to ensure that the practices and procedures of the Member States' health care systems are consistent with the principles and aims of the Code.[26] The UK government and the BMA support the principles and recommendations of the Code.

Global perspectives on child health

Although the current mortality and morbidity of infants and children in the UK are at their lowest levels ever recorded (see Chapter 3), there is still scope for improvement. The UNICEF under 5 years mortality rankings (1996) ranked the UK 18 ($n = 191$), with the mortality rate being seven per 1000 live births. Table 1.2 shows the top 18 countries and a random selection of those at the lower end.

The value of children is a social–psychological construct referring to the values attributed to children by parents, why they have children, and what they want from their children. Kagitcibasi reported on a study of the value of children which was conducted in nine countries (Indonesia, Germany, Korea, the Philippines, Singapore, Taiwan, Thailand, Turkey, and the USA) by comparing the motivations for child bearing of 20,000 married people. The several values attributed to children by parents could be grouped under three main value types:

- *Utilitarian* – the economic and material benefits of children both when they are young and when they grow up to be adults (offer old age security).
- *Psychological* – the fulfilment that children provide in terms of love, joy, pride, and companionship.
- *Social* – the general social acceptance that married adults gain when they have children and the desires for the continuation of the family.

The utilitarian value was stronger in less well developed countries. By contrast the psychological value was more prominent in more developed countries because children are not considered as economic assets, indeed they may be quite costly. The challenge is to move societies away from the utilitarian value to the psychological value, thereby reducing fertility with each child being valued in their own right.[27]

Table 1.2   Early childhood mortality rates

Ranking	Country	Mortality/1000 live births in children under 5 years
1	Sweden	4
1	Singapore	4
1	Finland	4
4	Switzerland	5
4	Spain	5
4	Ireland	5
7	Slovenia	6
7	Norway	6
7	Netherlands	6
7	Monaco	6
7	Japan	6
7	Germany	6
7	France	6
7	Denmark	6
7	Austria	6
7	Australia	6
7	Andorra	6
18	UK	7
18	Ireland	7
18	New Zealand	7
29	USA	8
43	Chile	13
99	Philippines	38
109	Turkey	47
146	India	111
159	Pakistan	136
191	Niger	320

(Source: UNICEF. *The State of the World's Children*. Oxford: Oxford University Press, 1998. By permission of Oxford University Press.)

Aim and scope of the report

This BMA report focuses specifically on the child, from conception to age 5, and on the impact of social and economic inequality on child health. For the purpose of the report "health" is defined as not simply the absence of ill health and disease but in a wider sense of developing a sense of "well-being", physically, emotionally, intellectually, psychologically, and spiritually.

Chapter 2 gives a brief overview of the key issues in child health today and Chapter 3 draws on the evidence of inequalities which are clearly apparent in child health within the UK at present. It also considers evidence regarding efficacy of interventions, in order that strategies can be employed to improve current and future health of children. Clearly the report cannot deal with all child health issues in depth, but a number of key issues were identified to illustrate inequity in child health, highlight the efficacy of certain interventions and point to the need for a total rather than service-orientated approach in addressing inequity and poor health and well-being in the early years of life.

The report will therefore consider issues relating to nutrition (Chapter 4), abuse and non-accidental injury (Chapter 5), disability (Chapter 6), and mental health/behavioural problems (Chapter 7).

Chapter 8 considers the origins of adult disease and how this may be programmed *in utero* and early childhood. Chapter 9 draws conclusions and presents a broad range of recommendations for actions that need to be taken, primarily outside of the NHS, if the UK is to provide an environment in which children are nurtured and their health in the early years of life recognised as key to the future health and well-being of the country.

This BMA policy report will be a valuable resource for doctors and all health care professionals working with children such as health visitors, members of the primary health care team, and paediatricians. Policy makers and workers involved in the health, education, social and voluntary sectors will also find this report a useful reference point in their work.

1 British Medical Association. *Complementary Medicine: new approaches to good practice.* London: BMA, 1993

2 British Medical Association. *Inequalities in Health.* London: BMA, 1995

3 British Medical Association. *Road Transport and Health.* London: BMA, 1997

4 British Medical Association. *Health and Environmental Impact Assessment: an integrated approach.* London: BMA, 1998

5 British Medical Association. *The Misuse of Drugs.* London: BMA, 1997

6 British Medical Association. *Domestic Violence: a health care issue?* London: BMA, 1998

7 British Medical Association. *Water: a vital resource.* London: BMA, 1994

8 British Medical Association. *Deprivation and Ill-health.* London: BMA, 1987

9 Department of Health. *The Health of the Nation.* London: HMSO, 1992

10 British Medical Association. *Strategies for National Renewal: a BMA commentary on the report of the Commission on Social Justice.* London: BMA, 1995

11 Department of Social Security. *Households Below Average Income (HBAI): a statistical analysis 1979-1992/93.* London: HMSO, 1995

12 Black D, Morris J, Smith C, *et al. Inequalities in Health: report of a research working group.* London: Department of Health and Social Security, 1980

13 Quick A, Wilkinson R. *Income and Health.* London: Socialist Health Association, 1991

14 Department of Health. *Independent Inquiry into Inequalities in Health*. London: The Stationery Office, 1998
15 The Prime Minister's Office. *The Government's Annual Report, 1997/8,* CM3969. London: The Stationery Office, 1998
16 Department of Health. *Our Healthier Nation: Green Paper,* CM3852. London: The Stationery Office, 1998
17 Department of Health. *Smoking Kills,* CM4177. London: The Stationery Office, 1998
18 Makins V. *Not Just a Nursery . . . multi-agency early years centres in action*. London: National Childrens Bureau, 1997
19 Chancellor of the Exchequer. *Modern Public Services for Britain: investing in reform. Comprehensive spending review: new public spending plans 1999–2002*. London: The Stationery Office, 1998
20 The Scottish Office. *Meeting the Child Care Challenge: a framework and consultation document*. London: The Stationery Office, 1998
21 Schaffer HR. *Making Decisions about Children: psychological questions and answers*. Oxford: Blackwell, 1990
22 Ruxton S. *Children in Europe*. London: NCH Action for Children, 1996
23 Department of Health. *The New NHS*. London: HMSO, 1997
24 *The United Nations Convention on the Rights of the Child*. Adopted by the General Assembly of the United Nations on 20 November 1989
25 World Medical Association. *Declaration of Ottawa, the right of the child to health care,* 17/170/E/Rev. Ottawa, Canada: 50th WMA General Assembly, 1998
26 WHO/UNICEF. *International Code of Marketing of Breastmilk Substitutes. Resolution WHA 34.22*. Geneva: World Health Organisation, 1981
27 Kagitcibasi C. The value of children: a key to gender issues. *International Child Health* 1998;**9**:15–24

Chapter 2 – Setting the scene

The level of civilisation attained by any society will be determined by the attention it has paid to the welfare of its children.

(Billy F Andrews MD, 1968)

Child population in the UK

In 1996, the total population of the UK was 58.8 million, an increase of 11% since 1961 (Figure 2.1). It is projected that this will increase to 60.7 million by 2031. Those under 16 years of age currently constitute 21% of the population, but it is predicted that this will decrease to 18% by 2021 with the increase in the population lying primarily with those aged 65 and over.[1] This is indicative of the declining birth rate and the increase in life expectancy. In 1995, the under 5 years age group totalled 3835,000 – 6.5% of the population. The estimate for 2031 is for a total of 3138,000 – 5.2% of the population.[2] The population structure is different in certain ethnic minority groups; for example, 20% of the white population in 1996–97 were under 16, compared to 38% of the Pakistani/Bangladeshi group.[3]

Fertility statistics

Fertility rates for older women have increased since the early 1980s, while those for younger women have declined (Figure 2.2). Since 1992 those in the 30–34 group have been more likely to give birth than those aged 20–24. The average age of a mother at the birth of her first child increased from 26.4 in 1976 to 28.6 in 1996.[1]

Family composition

The present family composition provides information on the situations in which children are living now and how this could change in the future. The average size of households in Britain has almost halved since the beginning of this century to 2.4 people per household in 1996–97; the increase in the number of households exceeded the growth in the population. The proportion of households comprising a "couple family" with dependent children has been in decline. In 1961, 38% of all households in Britain were of this type but by 1996–97 this had decreased to only 25%. There are clear differences in household structure in different regions and for different sections of the population. Although only one in 100 white or black ethnic group households comprised more than one family, for Indian and Pakistani/Bangladeshi households nearly one in ten households contained two or more families. In general, family size has reduced over the past 20 years influenced by a range of factors, including increased accessibility and provision of family planning services. In 1996–97 just over a quarter of dependent children lived in a family with three or more children.[1]

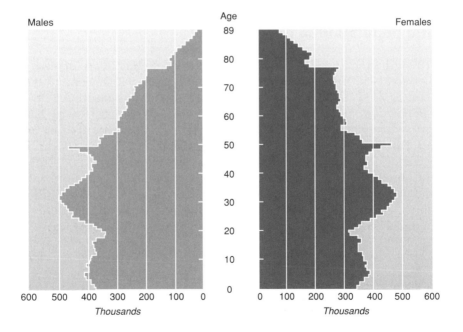

Fig 2.1 Population: by gender and age, 1996. (Source: Office for National Statistics, General Register Office for Scotland, Northern Ireland Statistics and Research Agency. In: Office for National Statistics. *Social Trends 28*. London: The Stationery Office, 1998. © Crown Copyright 1998)

The number of lone parent families has increased over the last 25 years. Lone parents headed around 21% of all families with dependent children in Britain in 1996, nearly three times the proportion in 1971. There was a gradual increase up until the mid-1980s as a result of divorce, while after 1986 a more rapid increase occurred because of the number of live births outside marriage. By far the majority of lone parent households are headed by women.[1] The British Household Panel Survey calculated that as a result of the forming of new partnerships half of all single parent mothers would have a duration of lone parenthood of 4 years or less.[4] The types of households children lived in in 1996–97 were as follows: 80% lived with a couple, 18% with a lone mother, and 2% with a lone father (Figure 2.3).[1]

In 1995 there were 155,000 divorces in England and Wales, affecting 160,000 children (around one in every 65 children).[1] The economic effects of divorce are undoubted. Now that most families depend on two incomes, splitting into two households inevitably reduces the money available to each

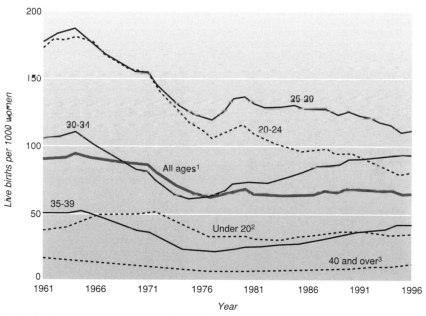

1 Total live births per 1000 women aged 15 to 44
2 Live births to women aged under 20 per 1000 women aged 15 to 19
3 Live births to women aged over 40 per 1000 women aged 40 to 44

Fig 2.2   Fertility rates: by age of mother at childbirth. (Source: Office for National Statistics, General Register Office for Scotland, Northern Ireland Statistics and Research Agency. In: Office for National Statistics. *Social Trends 28.* London: The Stationery Office, 1998. © Crown Copyright 1998)

15

and the possibility of reduced income or problems regarding child care may obviously have an effect upon children.

Of all live births in 1996, over a third were outside marriage. However, there is evidence to suggest that the majority of such births occur within a stable relationship. Four-fifths of such births were jointly registered by both parents in 1996. The teenage conception rate has decreased since the early 1990s and in 1995 for England and Wales stood at 59 per thousand 13–19 year olds. Fifty per cent of under 16 conceptions led to abortion in 1995.[1]

The expansion of the labour market for women has had an important effect for children in terms of child care. The number of women with children under the age of 5 years who are in the work force rose from 30% in 1985 to 43% in 1991 and will approach 50% by 2001. However, only a small minority were in full time employment.[5] Those working full time are primarily in career jobs and for the period 1990–92, 32% of professional or managerial women with a child under 5 worked full time whereas only 1% of mothers in unskilled occupations did.[6] The proportion of lone mothers with a child under age 5 who work outside the home, whether full or part time is much lower than the overall proportion of married mothers: 22% compared with 45%.[7] Parents, still especially mothers, are expected to take

Fig 2.3 Percentage of dependent children[1] living in different family types.

Great Britain   Percentages

	1972	1981	1986	1991–92	1996–97
Couple families					
1 child	16	18	18	17	17
2 children	35	41	41	37	37
3 or more children	41	29	28	28	26
Lone mother families					
1 child	2	3	4	5	5
2 children	2	4	5	7	7
3 or more children	2	3	3	6	6
Lone father families					
1 child	-	1	1	-	-
2 or more children	1	1	1	1	1
All dependent children	100	100	100	100	100

Source: General Household Survey, Office for National Statistics

[1]*1971 Census* – Dependent children: never–married children in families who were either under 15 years of age, or aged 15–24 and in full time education. *1991 Census* – Dependent children: never–married children in families who were either under 16 years of age, or aged 16–18 and in full time education. (Source: General Household Survey, Office for National Statistics. In: Office for National Statistics. *Social Trends 28*. London: The Stationery Office, 1998. © Crown Copyright 1999)

full responsibility for children's care, and to do so while earning. It is in this context that demands for purchased child care, for infants and toddlers as well as preschool children, have been increasing evermore rapidly since the early 1970s.[8]

In terms of social policy, we may therefore wish to focus on difficulties faced by lone parents, or working parents whose dual role of carer and provider can be particularly stressful. Lone parenthood is a risk factor for a child's health and lone parents are likely to need additional help and support. Clearly, then, policies which affect welfare provision and the labour market are important for child health issues.

Key health issues for children today

The major demographic, social, behavioural and medical developments which have occurred over this century have been reflected in the changes which have occurred in the health of the childhood population.[9] The most significant change in child health has been the rapid fall in deaths and morbidity from acute infections such as tuberculosis, measles, and whooping cough, which can be attributed to improvements in hygiene, living conditions, antibiotics, and immunisation. However, there is emerging evidence that the quality of children's health is being threatened by new problems of different types which relate to the effects of adverse demographic, economic and cultural developments;[9] for example, the increased prevalence of mental and emotional problems, asthma, and obesity. The World Health Organisation has projected that in the next 30 years, injury will overtake infectious disease as the major reason for global loss of healthy life years.[10]

Infant mortality

The Chief Medical Officer for England and Wales in his annual statement "On the State of the Public Health 1997" reported that the infant mortality rate had fallen to the lowest ever recorded with 5.9 babies dying per 1000 live births (Figure 2.4). In 1996, 3725 babies died before the age of 1 year, this fell to 3591 in 1997. During 1996 in England, there were 3345 stillbirths compared to 3250 in 1997. The stillbirth rate fell from 5.5 to 5.4 per 1000 total births between 1995 and 1996.[11] Worldwide, the infant mortality rate was 59 per 1000 live births in 1995.[10]

There has also been a large fall in recent years of postneonatal deaths, from 4.1 per 1000 live births in 1988 to 3.0 per 1000 in 1991. This has been almost entirely attributed to a fall in deaths from Sudden Infant Death Syndrome (SIDS).[9] In 1982, the mortality rate attributed to SIDS was 1.73 per 1000 live births, this declined to 1.25 in 1991.[9] SIDS, however, is still the largest single cause of infant death in the postneonatal period, accounting for 30% of all postneonatal deaths in England and Wales in 1992.[9]

Childhood mortality

Childhood mortality rates are at an historically low level and Figure 2.5 illustrates the main causes of childhood mortality by age and sex in England and Wales in 1991.

Injury and poisoning is the single commonest cause of death for boys of all ages outside infancy and for girls aged 5 and over. In 1991, cancer was the cause of 13% of deaths among children aged 1–4, although mortality from cancer has decreased over recent years. Congenital malformations account for almost one in five deaths under the age of 5. In 1971, child deaths due to diseases of the respiratory system were still a significant cause of mortality, accounting for 16.5% of child deaths; however, in 1991, this had declined to 8.5%.[9] Infectious diseases are much less likely to cause death and serious illness than at the turn of the century. In 1981, 15 children died of measles, in 1991, only one (Figure 2.6).[9]

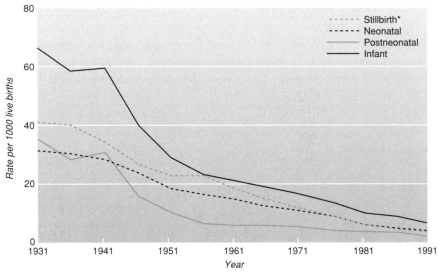

* Stillbirth rates per 1000 live + stillbirths

Fig 2.4 Stillbirth and infant mortality rates: 1931–91, England and Wales. (Source: Registrar General's Statistical Reviews 1931–73, OPCS Mortality Statistics – childhood 1974–91. In: Office of Population Censuses and Surveys. *The Health of Our Children: Decennial Supplement.* Series DS no 11. London: HMSO, 1995. © Crown Copyright 1999)

Trends in childhood morbidity

Over the past 20 years, there has been little change in the incidence of childhood cancers but between 1970 and 1985, hospital admissions for child cancer patients increased more than fourfold. However mortality rates have decreased slightly, which leads to the conclusion that improvements in treatment mean that children now survive for longer and many are cured.[9] The most common types of child cancer are leukaemia and brain tumours.

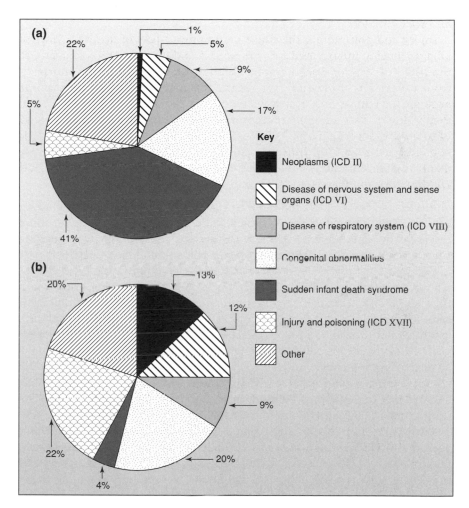

Fig 2.5   Main causes of childhood mortality by age and sex: 1991. (a) Postneonatal deaths: boys and girls (2106 deaths). (b) Deaths at ages 1–4: boys and girls (903 deaths). (Source: Mortality Statistics in Childhood, 1991. In: Office of Population Censuses and Surveys. *The Health of Our Children: Decennial Supplement*. Series DS No 11. London: HMSO, 1995. © Crown Copyright 1999)

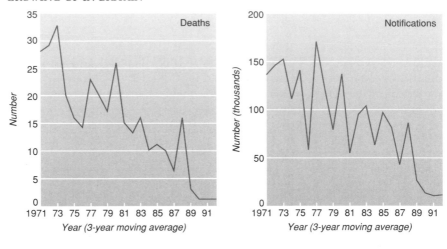

Fig 2.6 Deaths and notifications of measles: 1971–92, England and Wales. (Source: Communicable Disease Statistics 1982–92. In: Office of Population Censuses and Surveys. *The Health of Our Children: Decennial Supplement.* Series DS no 11. London: HMSO, 1995. © Crown Copyright 1999)

Considerable research is ongoing into possible causes of cancer, including genetic, environmental and chemical risk factors. For example, some research by Sir Richard Doll is underway, examining the possible correlation between electromagnetic radiation and childhood cancers.

Between 1987 and 1991, there was a 27% reduction in the incidence of whooping cough, with 5000 notifications in 1991. This has been attributed to a successful vaccination programme for the infection. Immunisation rates for all childhood infectious diseases have increased significantly in the last three decades. In the fourth quarter of 1997, 96% of children under 2 years of age were immunised against diphtheria, tetanus and polio, 94% against whooping cough, and 91% against measles.[12] Since 1988, when the measles, mumps, and rubella (MMR) vaccine was introduced, there has been a higher uptake of immunisation, which has in turn led to the notifications of measles falling to their lowest ever recorded levels.[1]

Adverse recent publicity suggesting a link between the MMR vaccine and autism and Crohn's disease seems to be leading to a fall in uptake which may in turn give rise to further measles deaths.[13] Promotion and presentation of vaccine policy to the public is very important, as many people may have inaccurate perceptions that some diseases no longer exist (for example tetanus) or that some diseases are trivial (for example measles and mumps).

While many of the infectious diseases encountered by children have been decreasing over recent decades, others have emerged and become of increasing importance. The notifications of meningococcal meningitis have been increasing over recent years. Between 1977 and 1984 there were 400–500 notifications per year, between 1990 and 1991, notifications were rising to over 1000 a year. Between 1987 and 1991, 68% of meningococcal infection notifications have been for children aged under 15 years, the rate being highest for babies aged less than 1 year.[9]

AIDS and HIV is also seen as an emerging infectious disease of concern to children's health in the UK. By the end of April 1998, a total of 334 cases of AIDS in children aged 14 years or under had been reported, of these 50% had died. Eighty-four per cent were infected by transmission from mother to infant, 10% by blood factor treatment (for example haemophilia), 5% by blood/tissue transfer, and 1% undetermined. A total of 817 children were reported infected with HIV by the end of April 1998, of whom 61% had acquired infection through mother to infant transmission. Of the 1234 children known to have been born to HIV infected mothers, 40% are known to be infected, 36% are known to be uninfected, and the status of the remaining 24% is undetermined at present.[14] There is now clear evidence, however, that transmission of HIV from an infected mother to her child can be greatly reduced by interventions such as antiretroviral treatment in pregnancy and in the perinatal period, and the avoidance of breastfeeding.[15]

Hospital admission rates for child injuries continue to rise, although it is not known whether this reflects a true increase in injury frequency or perhaps that thresholds for admission have changed.[9] It has been estimated that 2.33 million children attend an accident and emergency department annually and of these, approximately 5–10% require admission.[16] During 1987–89, 19% of 0–4 year olds consulted their family doctor following an accident.[17] The most common non–fatal accidents are road accidents, falls, and being struck with an object.

Respiratory disease remains a major cause of morbidity in children. Since the 1960s, hospital admissions of children aged 0 4 years with pneumonia have fallen but acute bronchitis admissions have increased.[9] Between 1991 and 1992, the Fourth General Practice Morbidity Survey found that 9.9% of boys aged 0–4 years and 7.2% of girls of the same age consulted their general practitioners for asthma at least once compared to 3.3% and 1.8% respectively between 1981 and 1982.[1] Hospital admissions for asthma have risen 13-fold since the early 1960s. From 1962 to 1985, there was an increase of 1300% for hospital admissions for asthma in the 0–4 year age group. In recent years, the annual increase has been around 20% for 0–4 year olds. Similar increases have occurred in most other developed countries.[9]

In 1997, the notification rate for live births with congenital abnormalities fell to 79.2 per 10,000 live births, 5% lower than in 1996 and 8% lower than in 1992.[11] Approximately 5% of all babies in England and Wales are born with a congenital malformation or other developmental defects such as Down's syndrome and spina bifida. The notification rate for central nervous system malformations has fallen by 52% over the 10 years between 1981 and 1991, 30% of this reduction has been attributed to prenatal detection and abortion. Folic acid supplementation has been shown to prevent 72% of neural tube defects in women who were at high risk of having a pregnancy with a neural tube defect.[9]

Fetal health

Action to improve fetal health clearly begins at the pre–conception stage, and ideally the problem of maternal smoking or drug consumption needs to be addressed well in advance of pregnancy. To tackle these problems effectively we need to understand the reasons why mothers may take up smoking or drug taking, and consider some of the interrelated issues such as poverty, unemployment and low self–esteem which may encourage a culture of substance abuse.

Pre–conception and health care

Proper preparation for conception is one of the most important methods for preventing birth defects.[18] It is important, for example, that women know about rubella immunisation before pregnancy. Complications to fetal health which may be caused by a rubella infection during pregnancy include deafness, pneumonitis, growth hormone deficiency, diabetes, ocular damage, vascular effects, and encephalitis.[19] Rubella is now part of the MMR vaccine. It is important to encourage the vaccination of children against childhood diseases but also to remember that mothers themselves may be at risk during pregnancy and the importance of adult immunisation should be made clear to all women who are planning a pregnancy.

The HEA's current folic acid campaign aims to encourage all women who hope to become pregnant to take a 400 μg supplement of folic acid and to increase their consumption of folate rich foods. An adequate intake of folic acid has been linked to a reduced risk of neural tube defects, low birthweight, and preterm delivery of infants. An evaluation of the HEA campaign based on the changing levels of public awareness of the benefits of folic acid, has shown that 49% of women surveyed in 1998 had unprompted recognition of the benefits of folic acid compared to 9% in 1995.[20]

Successful public health campaigns can therefore influence behaviour, although with multifactorial problems – such as smoking – we need also to tackle the wider issues of poverty and inequality. Women at the lower end of the socio–economic scale may once again be disadvantaged, and it is important that information – for example on the benefits of folic acid and rubella immunisation – should reach women through familiar media such as women's magazines as well as mainstream educational routes (from which some women will have been excluded). An effort should also be made to target ethnic minority women and women for whom English is a second language, so that they are made aware of these important health care issues.

Antenatal care

Screening for infections and birth defects during pregnancy is important for maximising child health both in the short and long term.

Screening is often offered as a routine part of antenatal care which can lead to being accepted unquestioningly and without due consideration. The provision of accurate and objective information is therefore particularly important for "routine screening". All tests that could identify fetal abnormality, or an increased risk of abnormality (including ultrasound scanning), need to be fully explained to the pregnant woman before she is asked to give consent.[21] The psycho-social side effects of screening are equally as important.

The BMA supports the view of the Royal College of Physicians who emphasised that the primary objectives of prenatal diagnosis are:

- to allow the widest possible range of informed choice to women and couples at risk of having children with an abnormality;
- to provide reassurance and reduce the level of anxiety associated with reproduction;
- to allow couples at risk to embark on having a family knowing that they may avoid the birth of seriously affected children through selective abortion;
- to ensure optimal treatment of affected infants through early diagnosis.[22]

In 1998, the NHS Executive wrote to all health authorities in England and Wales requesting them to ensure that all pregnant women be offered antenatal screening for hepatitis B, following a recommendation by the National Screening Committee. Health authorities have also been advised to ensure that all babies born to hepatitis B infected mothers receive a complete course of immunisation at birth.[23] Similarly, the Scottish Office Department of Health has requested that this be undertaken by all Scottish health boards.[24]

Sexually transmitted diseases, in particular syphilis, can have devastating effects on both the mother and the intra-uterine child and need to be detected and treated as early as possible in pregnancy through screening.[25]

HIV transmission from an infected mother to her child continues to be a problem in the UK. Comparing data from the Departments' Unlinked Anonymous Surveys with surveillance data on diagnosed infection in pregnant women and children shows that 70% of all HIV infections in pregnant women are not being clinically diagnosed before delivery.[26] An Inter-Collegiate Working Party consisting of representatives from the Royal College of Paediatrics and Child Health, the Royal College of Obstetricians and Gynaecologists, the Public Health Laboratory Service, the Faculty of Public Health Medicine, the Royal College of Physicians, the Royal College of Nursing, the Royal College of General Practitioners, the Royal College of Pathologists, and the Royal College of Midwives, has recently recommended that all pregnant women should receive information on HIV infection and its transmission and that HIV testing should be universally available in all antenatal clinics. It is recommended that testing for HIV should be integrated within established antenatal testing for infections such as hepatitis B, rubella, and syphilis. All tests should be used with the women's prior knowledge and verbal consent. There is clear evidence that transmission of HIV from an infected mother to her child can be greatly reduced by interventions such as antiretroviral treatment in pregnancy and in the perinatal period, and the avoidance of breastfeeding.[15]

The Royal College of Obstetricians and Gynaecologists has recently published a report highlighting the fact that domestic violence is a significant factor in perinatal mortality and morbidity compared to many other conditions that are routinely screened for. Violence during pregnancy is associated with premature birth, low birthweight babies and fetal injuries to limbs and organs as well as placental abruption and premature spontaneous rupture of the membranes.[27] Screening for domestic violence by health professionals should therefore be considered a priority and the recent publications from the BMA and the Royal College of General Practitioners consider how this may be achieved.[28, 29]

Smoking

The dangers of smoking during pregnancy are widely established,[30] it has been shown to reduce birthweight by an average of 200 g[31] and it is also associated with failure to thrive. Researchers have recently found that one of the strongest carcinogens (NNK) in tobacco smoke, which could cause potentially carcinogenic mutations, is transmitted to developing fetuses when a pregnant woman smokes.[32] Another study has concluded that exposure to maternal smoking during pregnancy may be an important risk factor in the development of attention deficit disorder and deficits in motor skills and perception. Social deprivation, language problems and clumsiness may also feature.[33] The use of tobacco during pregnancy is one of the most important risk factors for neonatal and late fetal death.[34, 35] Studies have concluded that maternal smoking during pregnancy doubles the risk of SIDS and household exposure to tobacco smoke has an independent additive effect.[36, 37]

Despite these known risks, a significant proportion of women continue to smoke in pregnancy and it is a particular problem for those who are young, unemployed, or from manual labour groups.[38] The "Infant Feeding Survey"[39] reported that mothers in 1995 were less likely than in 1990 to have smoked before pregnancy (35% compared with 38%) and were more likely to have given up smoking (33% compared with 27%). Hence mothers in the 1995 survey were less likely to have smoked during pregnancy (23% compared with 28% in 1990). The survey also compared smoking cessation rates in pregnancy by social class and found that at least 44% of mothers in non-manual groups who had smoked before pregnancy gave up smoking, compared with about 30% of mothers in social classes IV and V and 24% of mothers with no partner.[39] Overall in the UK in 1995, one-third of women smokers reported that they gave up smoking during pregnancy, which meets *The Health of the Nation*[40] target that at least one-third of women smokers should stop smoking at the start of their pregnancy by the year 2000. This still means, however, that the majority of women who smoke before pregnancy will continue to smoke at some level while they are pregnant.

There is evidence that maternal smoking during pregnancy can lead to babies being born with smaller lungs and airways than average, which would predispose them to respiratory illness and asthma.[31] Children exposed to passive smoking in the home also have increased risks of these problems.[41] It is almost impossible to distinguish between the independent contributions of prenatal and postnatal maternal smoking, although the increased risk associated with smoking by other household members suggests that exposure to environmental tobacco smoke after birth is a cause of acute chest illness in young children.[42] Parental smoking is clearly related to socio-economic status and is more common in poorer households. In 1990, 16% of women in professional households smoked cigarettes, compared with 38% of women in unskilled manual households.[43] In poorer households, limited space may expose children to the risks of passive smoking and inadequate heating and housing may pose additional risks to health.

Drugs and alcohol

Drinking alcohol and taking drugs can also have adverse effects on fetal health. The 1995 Infant Feeding Survey reports that of those women questioned, 66% drank while pregnant and 24% gave up completely during pregnancy.[39] Up to 2-3% of pregnant women are heavy drinkers during pregnancy and mothers with high alcohol consumption often have low intakes of protein, zinc, vitamin A, folic acid, and thiamine.[44] Alcohol may also trigger developmental abnormalities and miscarriage. The most serious but rare, consequence of maternal drinking can be Fetal Alcohol

Syndrome (FAS), which can result in delayed neurological development, growth impairment, and a variety of physical problems (for example, heart abnormalities and skeletal defects).[45] Women who drink heavily in pregnancy are also more likely to smoke and use illicit drugs[45] and are likely to suffer from multiple social disadvantage. The consumption of illegal drugs can lead to intra-uterine growth retardation. Maternal use of cocaine can lead to hypoxia of the fetus, resulting in possible brain damage, and an increased risk of SIDS.[46]

1 Office for National Statistics. *Social Trends 28.* London: The Stationery Office, 1998
2 Government Actuary's Department. *1994 National Population Projection.* London: HMSO, 1997
3 Office for National Statistics. *Social Trends 27.* London: HMSO, 1997
4 Gershuny J, Buck N, Coker O, *et al.* British Household Panel Survey. In: Office for National Statistics. *Social Trends 26.* London: HMSO, 1996
5 Office of Population Censuses and Surveys. *General Household Survey 1992.* London: HMSO, 1992
6 Joshi H, Macran S, Dex S. *Employment, Childbearing and Womens' Subsequent Labour Force Participation: Evidence from the British 1958 birth cohort, working paper.* London: Social Statistics Research Unit, City University, 1995
7 Monk S. From the margins to the mainstream: an employment strategy for lone parents. In: House of Commons Employment Committee. *Mothers in Employment, vol 3. Appendices to the Minutes of Evidence. First report (1994-95 session HC227).* London: HMSO, 1995
8 *Families, Children and Child Care. A major UK study of the effects of different kinds of care on children's development.* London: March, 1998
9 Office of Population Censuses and Surveys. *The Health of Our Children: decennial supplement.* Series DS no 11. London: HMSO, 1995
10 Director General of The World Health Organisation. *The World Health Report 1998. Life in the 21st century: a vision for all.* Geneva: WHO, 1998
11 Department of Health. *On the State of the Public Health: the Annual Report of the Chief Medical Officer of the Department of Health for the year 1997.* London: The Stationery Office, 1998
12 Public Health Laboratory Service. *CDR Weekly Report* 1998;**8**(13): 113–22
13 Public Health Laboratory Service. *CDR Weekly Report* 1998;**8**(39): 343–52
14 Public Health Laboratory Service. *CDR Weekly Report* 1998;**8**(30): 265–80
15 Royal College of Paediatrics and Child Health. *Recommendations of an Intercollegiate Working Party for Enhancing Voluntary Confidential HIV Testing in Pregnancy. Reducing mother to child transmission of HIV infection in the United Kingdom.* London: RCPCH, 1998
16 Kemp A, Sibert J. Childhood accidents: epidemiology, trends and prevention. *Journal of Accident and Emergency Medicine* 1997;**14**:316–20
17 Woodroffe C, Glickman M, Barker M, *et al. Children, Teenagers, Health: the key data.* Buckingham: Open University Press, 1993
18 Czeizel AE. Folic acid containing multivitamins and prevention of birth defects. In: Bendich A, Deckelbaum RJ, eds. *Preventive Nutrition: the comprehensive guide for health professionals.* Totowa, New Jersey: Humana Press, 1997
19 Hall AJ, Peckham CS. Infections in childhood and pregnancy as a cause of adult disease – methods and examples. In: Marmont MG, Wadsworth MEJ, eds. Fetal and early childhood environment: long–term health implications. *British Medical Bulletin* 1997;**53**(1):10–23
20 Health Education Authority. *Changing Preconceptions, vol 2. The folic acid campaign 1995–1998 research report.* London: HEA, 1998
21 British Medical Association. *Human Genetics. Choice and responsibility.* London: Oxford University Press, 1998
22 Royal College of Physicians. *Prenatal Diagnosis and Genetic Screening: community and service implications.* London: RCP, 1989

23 NHS Executive. *Screening of Pregnant Women for Hepatitis B and Immunisation of Babies at Risk*, HSC 1998/127. London: NHS Executive, 1998
24 Scottish Office Department of Health. *Screening of Pregnant Women for Hepatitis B and Immunisation of Babies at Risk*, HSC 1998/127. NHS MEL, 1998
25 Hurtig AK, Nicoll A, Carne C, *et al.* Syphilis in pregnant women and their children in the United Kingdom results from national clinician reporting surveys 1994–7. *British Medical Journal* 1998;**317**:1617–19
26 Department of Health. *Antenatal Testing for HIV. Better for your baby*, PL/CO (98)4 London: Department of Health, 1998
27 Bewley S, Friend J, Mezey G, eds. *Violence Against Women*. London: RCOG Press, 1997
28 Royal College of General Practitioners. *Domestic Violence: the general practitioner's role*. London: RCGP, 1999
29 British Medical Association. *Domestic Violence: a health care issue?* London: BMA, 1998
30 Royal College of Physicians. *Smoking and the Young*. London: RCP, 1992
31 Spencer N, Logan S. Smoking, socio–economic status and child health outcomes: the ongoing controversy. In: Spencer N, ed. *Progress in Community Child Health 2*. Edinburgh: Churchill Livingstone, 1998
32 Finette BA, O'Neill JP, Vacek PM, *et al.* Gene mutations with characteristic deletions in cord blood T lymphocytes associated with passive maternal exposure to tobacco smoke. *Nature Medicine* 1998;**4**:1144–51
33 Landgren M, Kjellman B, Gillberg C. Attention deficit disorder with developmental co–ordination disorders. *Archives of Disease in Childhood* 1998;**79**:207–12
34 Doll R, Gray R, Peto R, *et al.* Tobacco related diseases. *Journal of Smoking Related Diseases* 1994;**1**:3–13
35 Cnattingius S, Hagland B, Meirik O. Cigarette smoking as a risk factor for late fetal and early neo–natal death. *British Medical Journal* 1988;**297**:258–61
36 Anderson HR, Cook DG. Passive smoking and sudden infant death syndrome: review of the epidemiological evidence. *Thorax* 1997;**52**:1003–9
37 Blair PS, Fleming PJ, Bensley D, *et al.* Smoking and the sudden infant death syndrome: results from 1993–5 case–control study for confidential inquiry into stillbirths and deaths in infancy. *British Medical Journal* 1996;**313**(7051):195–8
38 Owen L, McNeill A, Callum C. Trends in smoking during pregnancy in England, 1992–7: quota sampling surveys. *British Medical Journal* 1998;**317**:728
39 Foster K, Lader D, Cheesebrough S. *Infant Feeding 1995*. London: HMSO, 1997
40 Department of Health. *The Health of the Nation*. London: HMSO, 1992
41 Upton M, Watt G, Davey Smith G, *et al.* Permanent effects of maternal smoking on offsprings' lung function. *Lancet* 1998;**352**:453
42 Strachan DP, Cook DG. Health effects of passive smoking 1. Parental smoking and lower respiratory illness in infancy and early childhood. *Thorax* 1997;**52**:905–14
43 Action on Smoking and Health. *Her Share of Misfortune: women, smoking and low income*. London: ASH, 1993
44 Strauss RS. Effects of intrauterine environment on childhood growth. In: Marmot ME, Wadsworth MEJ, eds. Fetal and early childhood environment: long–term health implications. *British Medical Bulletin* 1997;**53**(i):81–96
45 Royal College of Physicians. *Alcohol and the Young*. London: RCP, 1995
46 Nathanielsz PW. *Life Before Birth: the challenges of fetal development?* New York: WH Freeman, 1996

Chapter 3 – Inequalities in child health

The Chancellor has a much greater impact on health than the Secretary of State for Health, a thought that may well not cross the minds of either.

(Quick and Wilkinson, 1991)

Overall, the health of children in the UK is improving. However, national data can often obscure variations between regions, social classes and ethnic groups of people. These variations are important for the development of future health policies and programmes.

Common infectious diseases of childhood are coming under control through a combination of successful immunisation programmes, health promotion, disease prevention, and treatment. But, at the same time, the healthy growth and development of many children is threatened by economic and social influences and a decline in mortality is likely to be associated with an overall increase in morbidity. Clearly, even though mortality rates and morbidity rates for some diseases may be improving, others, such as respiratory problems, are rising and health inequalities between class groups in our society appear to be widening.

The landmark Black report[1] published in 1980 documented that despite the great improvements in the health of British people within the twentieth century, inequalities in health had persisted. Social class gradients were found to be present for many different causes of morbidity and mortality. The Black working party were in no doubt that although the health services may play a major role in determining the health of the nation, they could not on their own answer the challenge posed by the relationship between wide social inequalities and health. The evidence for the effect of both social and economic inequalities on health has grown since the Black report, and there is now a clearer explanation of the relationship and identification of key determinants of health. Despite this evidence, statistics reveal that inequalities within the UK are increasing rather than decreasing. The United Nations Development Programme considers that Britain is now one of the most unequal industrialised countries in the world.[2] In 1982 10% of the population had an income below half the national average, this rose to 20% by 1993 and has since fallen back to 19%.[3] Unskilled men have a mortality rate three times that of professional men.[4]

Poverty, poor housing, unemployment and smoking all clearly have effects on maternal and fetal health. Mothers (and their children) who are homeless face particular health challenges, which impact upon the child's birthweight and health in later life. For example, it was found that of mothers living in bed and breakfast accommodation in Hackney, 25% of their newborns had a birthweight below 2500 g, compared with 10% among babies of local area residents, and 7.2% in England.[5] Poor housing can also affect maternal health by contributing to depression, higher rates of respiratory infection, poor nutrition (many homeless women staying in bed and breakfast accommodation do not have access to a kitchen), and an increased risk of smoking, alcoholism or drug abuse.

Definitions of disadvantage

There are difficulties with the measures used to categorise individuals into groups that relate to their level of deprivation.[6] Social class is a widely used measure, however this is not necessarily an indicator of "material" wealth that is, housing, adequate income, etc. Material disadvantage may be absolute, relative, or both. Children and other family members are classified according to the occupation of the main earner in the family. Occupation is therefore used as a proxy measure of income. Social class is perhaps becoming a poorer measure of socio-economic status than in the past, as home ownership, second incomes, single parenthood and unemployment cut across the traditional relationship between husband's occupation and family resources. Using class-based analysis excludes people classified as unoccupied, for example, economically inactive single mothers.[7] This group are a high risk group for living in poverty as well as experiencing relatively high risks of child mortality. The longitudinal studies of the Office of Population Censuses and Surveys (OPCS)[8] have demonstrated the value of other measures of social and economic circumstances, such as housing tenure and car ownership. These have been found to be more effective discriminators of mortality differences than social class and do not exclude economically inactive people.

For children it is not solely material wealth that matters and their well-being is directly related to their emotional environment. However materially privileged a child's family is, problems will arise if they are unwanted or resented, neglected or abused. Poverty, unemployment or homelessness may exert their effect on the child by the overall reduction in parental capacity to meet their own and their children's emotional needs. With regard to children, social disadvantage is therefore probably best considered in terms of the quality of child care. Good child care involves a mutually affectionate relationship based on respect, empathy and genuineness with one or preferably more adults, consistent discipline based on positive reward for good behaviour rather than punishment for bad, and intellectual stimulation appropriate to the child's level of development.

Socio-economic inequalities and health

The OPCS report *The Health of Our Children*[9] and the Office for National Statistics (ONS) report *Health Inequalities*[10] have reviewed data for childhood mortality and morbidity and have drawn a number of key points from the data.

- During the 1980s and early 1990s infant and childhood mortality rates fell for all social classes, but the social class differentials persisted. In 1993-95 the infant mortality rate for social class V births was 70% higher than that of social class I births.
- Babies born weighing under 2500 g in 1991 accounted for 59% of neonatal deaths. In 1994 in England and Wales the average birthweight in social class V was 115 g lighter than in social class I for births inside marriage and 130 g lighter for births outside marriage registered by both parents.
- In 1993 the Children's Dental Health Survey found that among 12 year olds 45% from non-manual households suffered from any form of decay, compared to 68% from unskilled manual households.
- Childhood mortality from injury and poisoning fell between the early 1980s and early 1990s for all social classes. However the differential between the classes increased as a result of the smaller decline occurring in social classes IV and V as compared to social classes I and II.

Social classes

Children in manual social class families are likely to have more illnesses than those in non-manual social class families. Children are categorised to a social class relating to that of the head of their household. At all ages in childhood there is a gradient of risk of increased mortality with increasing social disadvantage, most marked at ages 1-4 years.[9] Boys are consistently at higher risk than girls. Although there has been a significant decline in infant mortality as a whole, the gap between classes remains substantial. Nine per 1000 babies born in social class V were stillborn or died in the first week of life, compared with six per 1000 babies born in social class I. For deaths in the first year of life this was eight per 1000 for social class V compared to five per 1000 babies in social class I.[11] The role of unequal societies in the health of children is also revealed by examining the relative poverty in different countries and the infant mortality rates. The Organisation for Economic Co-operation and Development (OECD) figures reveal a direct relationship between the percentage of the population in relative poverty and the infant mortality rate.[12] A study by Mcisaac and Wilkinson of the income distribution for the 13 OECD countries found that a more egalitarian distribution of income was related to lower all-cause mortality rates in both sexes in most age groups.[13]

Other indicators of inequality in health for children are accident rates, with children in social class V four times more likely to suffer accidental death than those in social class I. For deaths from fires or flames the ratio of social class I to V is 1:9.[14] Although there has been a decline in death rates from injury and poisoning for children of all classes, the decrease has been greater for those in higher social classes. Socio-economic inequalities in child injury death rates have therefore increased.[15] Children aged 0-15 with a father in social class V have 1.85 times the rate of limiting longstanding illness than those in social class I.[16] In addition, children's development in terms of birthweight and height at primary school age is worse in deprived areas.[17]

The factors operating to cause such wide differences in morbidity and mortality between social classes obviously need to be identified if action is to be taken to improve the current situation. However, the explanation for the relationship is still far from clear and a number of theories have developed. The favoured explanation in recent years has emphasised different patterns of risk factor accumulation by social position, that is "factors that combine and accumulate over the life course".[18] It is clear that from the time they are born, young children have a very different experience of factors hazardous to their health. An individual's chance of experiencing multiple health risks throughout life is influenced powerfully by social position.[19]

There is clear evidence of the importance of a "healthy" environment in the early years in order to protect current health and prevent future ill health. One factor that cannot be overlooked in providing a "healthy" environment is an adequate income. Although poverty is not the only factor that may lead to adverse outcomes for individuals, it is a factor that exacerbates and contributes to many other risk factors and could be said to be the biggest risk of all.

Definitions of poverty

Poverty can be defined in a number of different ways. A constant or fixed poverty level, that is "absolute" poverty, may be used, as may "relative" poverty that reflects levels of income in comparison to the majority of the population. Relative poverty more accurately reflects the situation for

31

individuals in today's society, as by utilising measures of absolute poverty there is an assumption that standards of living and our notions of what is essential or necessary do not change and adapt over time. There are two key sources of statistics relating to children's experience of poverty: Low Income Families (LIF)[20, 21] and Households Below Average Income (HBAI).[22] Both of these sets of data are derived from an annual government survey of around 7000 households in the UK. The LIF statistics establish the poverty line by reference to the level of income support, with poverty being defined as having an income equivalent to or below the relevant income support level. For example, for a couple with two children aged under 11 years, the 1995/96 level would be £115.15 a week or less. The LIF reveals that in 1979 14% of the population were living in poverty but this increased to 24% by 1992. The statistics show that it is couples with children who account for most of the increase between 1979 and 1992 of people living below supplementary benefit/income support levels. The LIF indicates that in 1992, 29% of all children were living in poverty; 6% of all children were living below the poverty line.

Poverty and family composition

The risk of falling into poverty depends on the type of family. In 1992 78% of children growing up in lone parent families were living in poverty compared to 18% of children in two parent families. For adolescent or school-age mothers the risk is great as pregnancy is a common reason for non-completion of schooling with the consequent risks of unemployment. A key reason for the numbers of individuals living below the poverty line is that many are not taking up the means tested benefits to which they are entitled. It is estimated that around £2 billion of means tested benefits went unclaimed in 1992, although the breakdown of the groups of population to which it refers is unknown.[23] For some individuals, they may only be able to earn a low income which is less, or little more than the social security benefits to which they are entitled. This can create an ethos of social security dependence, an attitude of mind to influence children and perpetuate a feeling of failure and inferiority. It is unlikely that the level of minimum wage so far discussed will materially affect the situation and the poverty trap will continue to exist.

The HBAI statistics examine the living standards of people earning 50% or less of the average income within England and Wales. This level of income when compared to the average is frequently used as a measure of the poverty line. The statistics reveal unemployment as a crucial cause of poverty, accounting for more than a fifth of those in poverty. With regard to family status, couples with children account for the largest group in poverty

(37%), the next largest group is lone parents who make up 17% of those in poverty. It is useful to consider the risk of falling into poverty by family status. The risk is highest for lone parents at 58%, for couples with children it is 24% as opposed to 13% for couples without children. The risk for couples with children tripled between 1979 and 1992/93. It is therefore evident that having children increases the risk of falling into poverty quite significantly.

The HBAI statistics also show an increase in the proportion of children living in poverty. In 1979 10% of all children lived in poverty, this had risen to 33% of all children in 1992/93, a rise of 36%. There is a higher proportion of children living in poverty (33%) than the population as a whole (25%). Children are therefore disproportionately affected by poverty. Twenty-nine per cent of all children living in poverty live in a family where there is one or more full time workers; 71% of all children living in poverty live in a family where there is no full time worker - this group of children constitutes those at greatest risk of poverty.

The figures used to define poverty could be assumed to define an adequate income, however, measures of income have been utilised to reveal the shortfall between the defined levels and the needs of families. One measure used is the modest but adequate budget (MAB).[24] Items are included in the budget if more than half the population have them or they are regarded as necessities in public opinion surveys. For example a week's annual holiday in the UK is included but holidays abroad are not, the costs of spectacles are not included but the costs of sight tests are. When such comparisons are made for a couple with two children living on the poverty line as defined by income support, the poverty line only provides 39% of the MAB. With the definition of poverty based on 50% of average income, only 54% of the MAB is covered.

Parenting itself can be considered as creating inequity, as parenting imposes enormous economic and practical burdens that are inequitably born by mothers. It has been estimated that having a child reduces a woman's average lifetime earnings (and pension) by two-thirds, whether she takes time out of work to care for that child herself or money out of her wage or salary to pay someone else to do so. The pay gap between women and men is largely a result of family responsibilities. The earnings of single childless women, on average, are 95% of those of single childless men; but married mothers earn, on average, only 60% of the pay of married fathers. The composite costs of raising a child have been estimated at between £50,000 and £80,000 in the UK and detailed budgets show that it cost an average of around £3000 per year to keep a child in Britain at just above poverty level.[25-28]

It is clear that large numbers of children are living on less than adequate incomes and that it is families and particularly single parents who are most at risk of falling into poverty. There is therefore a need to focus attention on mechanisms by which to reduce the financial and other risks for those with children.

Reducing inequalities in health

There is substantial evidence that a number of factors influence health in the early years of life and that these factors may also affect health in later life. This fact is now undisputed. There is, however, less evidence available on effective interventions that may be utilised to prevent ill health and to reduce inequity. It is in this area that future policy must now concentrate.

The evidence that is available can be utilised to predict what is likely to succeed where there is no direct evidence of efficacy. A comprehensive approach to this problem is likely to be required and interventions are therefore needed in areas other than health services. Intervention studies in the early years suggest that performance in two basic domains of child development, the cognitive and the social-emotional (education and parenting), can be modified in ways which should improve long-term outcomes.[29] Interestingly, the interventions identified for particular problems do in many cases have beneficial effects for a range of problems, and can therefore be said to be of benefit more generally for the health and well-being of many young children. Responsibility for the interventions identified cuts across the remit of many organisations and government departments and it is therefore clear that any successful intervention will need a multisectoral approach.

There are many interventions that could protect against inequalities both generally and in health. Some interventions have been more robustly evaluated than others. Inevitably, not all projects and services will have the time, money and expertise to evaluate the impact of their work on children's health in sophisticated ways. This report does not exclude projects which do not include rigorous evaluations of effectiveness of the sort described above. Many projects may not collect specific outcome data relating to children's health, and yet on theoretical grounds are highly likely to have a beneficial impact on family well-being. Projects of this sort are also considered, and where evidence of effectiveness has been demonstrated more substantially, this is highlighted.

In terms of factors that could protect against inequalities, the Carnegie Task Force on meeting the needs of young children concluded that the following could be considered "protective" in early years:

- *Temperament and perinatal factors* (such as full-term birth and normal birthweight): having characteristics that attract and encourage care-giving.
- *Dependable caregivers:* growing up in a family with one or two dependable adults whose child rearing practices are positive and appropriate.

- *Community support:* living in a loving, supportive and safe community can limit the risk to health.

Generally, it appears that educational interventions and family support offer the best means yet of protecting children from inequalities and therefore for protecting their health. Support can take several different guises, it can be interpersonal or emotional, practical (child care or safe environments), or financial. There is now a considerable body of experimental knowledge which suggests that the effectiveness of interpersonal "support" depends on the supporter's capacity to enable parents to feel less isolated, less criticised, and less vulnerable. So whether the support is effective depends upon the interpersonal skill of the person doing the support, on working in a way which is accepting, encouraging, valuing, and empowering.

Educational interventions

The key qualities are those which have been defined as the key qualities of the therapeutic relationship - respect, empathy, and genuineness.[30] Studies have concluded that parental help has provided significant advantage to children in educational attainment and that such children as adults were more likely to be enthusiastic about their own children's education. Early educational initiatives have been the subject of scrutiny and information is available upon their efficacy. The most well known and researched programme is Head Start.

Head Start is an American project aimed at breaking "the cycle of poverty". The programme received government funding for over 20 years. Early studies of the programme that only examined intelligence found that the benefits of taking part in the programme were lost on entry to school. However, when a broader range of outcome measures were used benefits for the programme were identified in cognitive ability, self-esteem, scholastic achievement, motivation, and social behaviour.[31] These benefits were however not maintained throughout later school years. Studies that have utilised long follow-up periods have also been carried out and a meta-analysis of these found that there was a strong correlation between good cognitively oriented preschool programmes and later school competence. Those interviewed at 19 years of age were generally more achievement oriented and less likely to be in "special" education.[32] Follow-up is continuing and good effects continue to be shown. In the Republic of Ireland, one study showed that early-years education had positive effects that lasted well beyond the primary school years and affected much more than children's academic performance.[33]

In a further study in the USA of the High Scope programme, researchers monitored and costed the effect of preschool education for children from poor families and the study followed up the individuals until they were 29 years of age.[34] Those who had preschool education were considerably more likely to complete high school or further education, three times more likely to own their own homes, four times more likely to earn a good income and five times less likely to have been in repeated trouble with the law. It was estimated that every $1 invested in nursery education led to a saving of $7 on police, prisons, probation services, and the payment of taxes by individuals now in employment. The benefits of preschool education such as improving income and housing will ultimately have an impact on health.

A good general education which covers an overall programme of personal, social and health education or "life preparation" appears to help young women to avoid early pregnancy, to avoid taking up smoking, and also to help them cease smoking in pregnancy. Sex education should be embedded in this overall education programme.[35] Studies have shown that well designed sex education programmes can have desirable effects, such as delaying the age of first intercourse or encouraging the use of condoms or other forms of contraception.[36-38] A review of the means of preventing and reducing the adverse effects of unintended teenage pregnancies concluded that school based sex education can be effective in reducing teenage pregnancy, especially when linked to access to contraceptive services. The most reliable evidence showed that sex education did not increase sexual activity or pregnancy rates.[39] Some common features of effective programmes have been identified, including the use of participatory teaching methods which enable pupils to be actively involved in their learning so as to personalise information and address social pressures. "Abstinence" programmes have not been shown to be effective.[35]

Family support

In terms of psychological health, prenatal and infant development programmes have been assessed, with most programmes consisting of home visiting of at-risk families.

One programme in the USA, which started in 1977, provided nurse visiting to 400 women, 85% of whom were either on a low income, unmarried, or teenaged. These women were visited regularly from pregnancy until their child was 2, with an average of nine visits in pregnancy and 23 visits in the subsequent 2 years. The nurses aimed to develop close therapeutic relationships with the mothers, within which they promoted sensitive responsive caregiving, encouraged the use of social support and formal child support services, and developed the mothers' sense of self-efficacy. The mothers were also offered free transport to health care facilities and screening for health care problems. The programme was evaluated in a randomised controlled trial against a group offered no intervention, and another group offered free transport and health screening alone. Many positive effects were demonstrated, including a substantially lower rate of child abuse and neglect among the poor unmarried teens who received the service (4% compared to 19% in the control group), fewer accident and emergency visits, and home environments more conducive to their intellectual and emotional development.[40] A further comprehensive family support project studied economically disadvantaged adolescent first time mothers, from birth of their child to 30 months, with long-term follow-up. In the short- and long-term follow-up measures of educational achievement showed benefits for those in the programme.[41] A review of a number of assessed programmes found both short- and long-term benefits where programmes were of long duration, were begun prenatally, and had home visits as a major component. Short-term effects included better physical health, better nutrition, fewer low birthweight babies, fewer accident and emergency visits, fewer feeding problems, and reduced incidence of child abuse. Long-term benefits included less aggressiveness and distraction in schools, less delinquency, better attitudes toward school, and better social functioning.[42] A systematic review of randomised controlled trials examined the effect of home visiting in childhood injury prevention.[43] Again it was concluded that home visiting programmes have the potential to reduce significantly the rates of childhood injury. It was not possible to estimate the effect on child abuse, as reported abuse could not be used as a valid outcome measure because of the differential surveillance for child abuse between intervention and control groups.

The efficacy of social support has also been shown through programmes in the UK. The Child Development Programme offered monthly professional support visits to all new parents, antenatally and for the first year of life. Emphasis was placed on the health and well-being of the mother as a person with her own interests and future. Parents were encouraged to set tasks to carry out with their children in the month following the visit. Evaluation indicated that despite programme families being more disadvantaged than non-programme families on nearly all outcome measures, programme families scored higher than non-programme. In addition, for the programme families there was a lower rate of registration on the Child Protection Register and a lower rate of physical abuse.[44] Other interventions have involved mature non-professional volunteer women supporting new mothers. The intervention was successful by a number of measures such as immunisation uptake, nutrition, continuation of breastfeeding, and constructive play between parent and child.[45] Social support for women at risk of low birthweight babies has also proven successful.[46] Measures to reduce the income gap have also proven effective in improving birthweight. A randomised controlled trial on income maintenance shows that a guaranteed minimum income to pregnant women in low income families was associated with a significant increase in birthweight in the intervention group.[47]

Interventions designed to reduce the incidence of child abuse and neglect have shown some success and a review of a number of interventions concluded that long-term visitation had been shown to be effective in the prevention of child physical abuse and neglect among families with one or more of single parenthood, poverty, and teenage parent status. The evidence regarding short-term home visitation, early and extended post-partum contact, intensive paediatric contact, use of drop-in centre, classroom education and parent training was found to be inconclusive.[48]

It has been suggested that behavioural and cognitive-behavioural methods are ahead of other interventions in respect of effective prevention work.[30] Parent training to enable parents to manage their children's behaviour, reduce conflict and confrontation while increasing compliance, co-operation and pleasant interaction and to favour reward rather than punishment in terms of discipline has had a positive effect with a range of child behaviour problems.[49,50] However, there are wide variations in the content and delivery of such programmes and there are a number of families with particular problems for whom the approach is unlikely to be successful.[30] Anger control strategies have also been utilised and evaluated on the basis that it is not feelings or impulses of anger that distinguish between abusive and non-abusive families but the ability to control those feelings. The efficacy of anger control training has not been demonstrated in the same way as parent training.[51] Family therapy approaches have also been evaluated, but again the research suffers from the wide range of types of therapy used for different family structures and problems, making much of the data non-comparable.[30]

The evidence is indicative of the need for long-term personal contact with at-risk families. Such interventions are likely to be costly and it would be useful to establish their cost benefits in the long term if they are to be promoted nationally. Certain interventions have been costed and been shown to be cost effective. For example, it has been estimated that care for a preterm baby, needed for anywhere from 3 to 60 days, costs approx-imately $3000 per day. However, rates of premature birth are reduced by adequate antenatal care, which costs around $600 per pregnancy. The US Institute of Medicine of the National Academy of Sciences calculates that the extra cost of increasing the availability and accessibility of antenatal care sufficiently to reduce the numbers of babies born preterm by 2–3% would lead directly to savings of at least three times its magnitude.[52] The costs of long–term measures to prevent child abuse and neglect are difficult to calculate, but even when a child's removal from the home is imminent or otherwise inevitable short–term intensive casework can render it unneces-sary and although expensive it is highly cost effective. An American programme Homebuilders, cost $2600 per family compared to $3600 per annum per child for foster care and up to $67,000 per annum for institutional care. At the end of 1 year, 90% of the children were still with their families. The savings for that year were calculated to amount to at least three times the otherwise inevitable expenditure.[53] As stated by the Committee on Economic Development: "improving the prospects for disadvantaged children is not an expense but an excellent investment, one that can be postponed only at much greater cost to society".

1 Black D, Morris J, Smith C, *et al*. *Inequalities in Health: report of a research working group.* London: Department of Health and Social Security, 1980
2 United Nations Development Programme. *Human Development Report 1996.* New York: Oxford University Press, 1996
3 Office for National Statistics. *Social Trends 27.* London: HMSO, 1997
4 Drever F, Whitehead M, Roden M. Current patterns and trends in male mortality by social class (based on occupation). In: Office of Population Censuses and Surveys. *Population Trends.* London: HMSO, 1996
5 Parsons L. Homeless families in Hackney. *Public Health* 1991;**105**:287–96
6 British Medical Association. *Deprivation and Ill–health.* London: BMA, 1987
7 Judge K, Benzeval M. Health inequalities: new concerns about the children of single mothers. *British Medical Journal* 1993;**306**:677–80
8 Goldblatt P. *Longitudinal Study: mortality and social organisation 1971–81.* OPCS series LS no 6. London: HMSO, 1990
9 Office of Population Censuses and Surveys. *The Health of Our Children: decennial supplement.* Series DS no 11. London: HMSO, 1995
10 Office for National Statistics. *Health Inequalities: decennial supplement.* Series DS no 15. London: ONS, 1997
11 National Children's Home Action for Children. *Factfile 1996/97.* London: NCH, 1996
12 Wennemo I. Infant mortality, public policy and inequality – a comparison of 18 industrialised countries 1950–85. *Sociological Health and Illness* 1993;**15**:429–46
13 Mcisaac SJ, Wilkinson RG. Income distribution and cause specific mortality. *European Journal of Public Health* 1997;**7**:45 53
14 Office of Population Censuses and Surveys. *Child Accident Statistics 1993.* London: OPCS, 1994
15 Roberts I, Power C. Does the decline in child injury mortality vary by social class? A comparison of class specific mortality in 1981 and 1991. *British Medical Journal* 1996;**313**:784–6
16 Office of Population Censuses and Surveys. *General Household Survey 1993.* London: HMSO, 1995
17 Reading R, Raybould S, Jarvis S. Deprivation, low birthweight and children's height: a comparison between rural and urban areas. *British Medical Journal* 1993;**307**:1458–62
18 Blane D, Bartley M, Smith GD. Disease aetiology and materialist explanations of socio–economic mortality differentials. *European Journal of Public Health* 1997;**7**:385–91
19 Power C, Matthews S. Origins of health inequalities in a national population sample. *Lancet* 1997;**350**:1584–9
20 Social Security Committee. *Low Income Statistics: low income families (LIF) 1979–89. First Report.* London: HMSO, 1993
21 Social Security Committee. *Low Income Statistics: low income families (LIF) 1989–1992. Second Report.* London: HMSO, 1995
22 Department of Social Security. *Households Below Average Income (HBAI): a statistical analysis 1979–1992/93.* London: HMSO, 1995
23 Department of Social Security. *Income–related Benefits: estimates of take–up in 1992.* London: HMSO, 1995
24 Family Budget Unit. *Modest but adequate: summary budgets for sixteen households, October 1994 prices.* York: Family Budget Unit, 1995
25 Joshi H. The cost of caring. In: Glendenning C, Miller J, eds. *Women and Poverty in Britain in the 1990s.* London: Wheatsheaf, 1992

26 Hewlett SA. *Child Neglect in Rich Nations*. New York: UNICEF, 1993
27 Oldfield N, Yu ACS. *The Cost of a Child*. London: Child Poverty Action Group, 1993
28 Rock A. Can you afford your kids? *Money* 1990;**19**:88–99
29 Hertzman C, Wiens M. Child development and long–term outcomes: a population health perspective and summary of successful interventions. *Social Science and Medicine* 1996;**43**:1083–95
30 Macdonald G, Roberts H. *What Works in the Early Years? Effective interventions for children and their families in health, social welfare, education and child protection*. London: Barnardos, 1995
31 McKey HR, Condelli L, Ganson H, *et al*. *The Impact of Head Start on Children, Families and Communities*. Washington DC: The Head Start Bureau, 1985
32 Lazar I, Darlington R. Lasting effects of early education: a report from the consortium for longitudinal studies. *Monographs of the Society for Research in Child Development* 1982;**47**:2–3
33 Kellaghan T, Greaney BJ. *The Education and Development of Students Following Participation in a Pre–school Programme in a Disadvantaged Area in Dublin*. Studies and Evaluation Paper No 12. The Hague: Bernard van Leer Foundation, 1993
34 Schweinhart L, Barnes H, Weikart D. *The High Scope Perry Preschool Study through Age 27*. Michigan: High Scope Press, 1993
35 British Medical Association. *School Sex Education: good practice and policy*. London: BMA, 1997
36 Kirby D, Short L, Collins J, *et al*. School based programs to reduce sexual risk behaviours: a review of effectiveness. *Public Health Reports* 1994;**109**:339–60
37 Kirby D. Sex and HIV/AIDS education in schools. *British Medical Journal* 1995:**311**:403
38 Oakley A, Fullerton D, Holland J, *et al*. Sexual health education interventions for young people: a methodological review. *British Medical Journal* 1995:**310**:158–62
39 NHS Centre for Reviews and Dissemination. Preventing and reducing the adverse effects of unintended teenage pregnancies. *Effective Health Care* 1997;**3**:1–12
40 Olds DL, Henderson CR, Chamberlin R, *et al*. Improving the delivery of prenatal care and outcomes of pregnancy: a randomised trial of nurse home visitation. *Pediatrics* 1986;**77**:16–27
41 Seitz V, Apfel N, Rosenbaum L, *et al*. Long–term effects of projects Head Start and Follow Through: the New Haven Project. In: Consortium for Longitudinal Studies. *Lasting Effects of Preschool Programs*. New Jersey: Lawrence Erlbaum, 1983
42 Ministry of Community and Social Services. *Better Beginnings, Better Futures: an integrated model of primary prevention of emotional and behavioural problems*. Ontario: Queens Printer for Ontario, 1989
43 Roberts I, Kramer MS, Suissa S. Does home visiting prevent childhood injury? A systematic review of randomised controlled trials. *British Medical Journal* 1996; **312**:29–33
44 Barker WE, Anderson RA, Chalmers C. *Health Trends over Time and Major Outcomes of the Child Development Programme*. Belfast: Eastern Health and Social Services Board, Bristol ECDU, 1994
45 Johnson Z, Howell F, Molloy B. Community mothers' programme: randomised controlled trial of non–professional intervention in parenting. *British Medical Journal* 1993;**306**:1449–52
46 Oakley A, Rajan L, Grant A. Social support and pregnancy outcome. *British Journal of Obstetrics and Gynaecology* 1990;**97**:155–62
47 Kehrer BH, Wolin CM. Impact of income maintenance on low birthweight: evidence from the Gary experiment. *Journal of Human Resources* 1979;**14**:434–62
48 MacMillan HL, MacMillan JH, Offord DR, *et al*. Primary prevention of child physical abusc and neglect. A critical review: part 1. *Journal of Child Psychology and Psychiatry and Allied Professions* 1994;**35**:835–56
49 Miller GE, Prinz RJ. Enhancement of social learning family interventions for childhood conduct disorders. *Psychological Bulletin* 1990;**108**:291–307
50 Dumas JE. Treating anti–social behaviour in children: child and family approaches. *Clinical Psychology Review* 1989;**9**:197–222

51 Barth RP, Blythe BJ, Schinke SP, *et al*. Self control training with maltreating children. *Child Welfare* 1983;4:313–24
52 Institute of Medicine of the National Academy of Sciences. *Preventing Low Birthweight*. Washington DC: National Academy Press, 1985
53 Behavioural Sciences Institute. *Homebuilders Programme*. Washington DC: BSI, 1987

Chapter 4 – Nutrition

Sometimes when my son has said to me he's hungry, I just feel very desperate and alone, and a bit of a failure I suppose.

(A parent, 1996)

The nutritional needs of children aged 0–5 years

The years between 0 and 5 are demanding for the developing child; years in which they acquire many physical, social and psychological structures for life and learning. Unfortunately, many British 0–5 year olds are not being aided in these tasks by good nutrition: the problem is most acute for those children who are born into and live their early years in poverty.

The diet of the early years of life needs to be relatively more "nutrient dense" than the middle years. This is because the physical requirements for nutrients must be met within a relatively small number of calories and generally small quantities of food. Dietary guidelines are generally applied to the older children and adult population, and some commentators have noted that little is known about the appropriateness of these dietary recommendations for children, particularly during the preschool years.[1]

There is no doubt about the health benefits of breastfeeding during early infancy. Continued breastfeeding is therefore recommended throughout the first year of life. However neither breastmilk nor formula can supply all the nutritional needs of the infant during the second 6 months of life.

Weaning begins when semi–solid food starts to be given in addition to milk starting between the ages of 3 and 6 months. The weaning period is not only important because of the need to introduce nutritional variety and replenish iron stores; it is also a critical period within which to introduce and accustom infants to the experience and taste of different foods. There may be an important imprinting function, making this the ideal time to introduce particular foods such as vegetables and fruits. There is evidence that food preferences developed during these years may affect food preference behaviour throughout life.[2]

The nutritional status of British 0–5 year olds

Unfortunately many British children are given inappropriate weaning foods, including sweet and salty foods such as crisps, sweets, soft drinks, etc. A diet high in these foods induces higher blood pressures within 6 months; dental erosions of primary teeth begin; and harmful dietary patterns for life are established.[3] If the diet is insufficiently nutrient dense then the suboptimal vitamin and mineral intake may affect immune function. This may contribute to the predisposition among children from lower socio–economic groups to recurrent infections.

General trends in diets show that for children from lower socio–economic groups:

- more foods are consumed out of the home;
- more processed foods are consumed;
- snacking and snack foods are contributing greater proportions of energy to the diet.

Dietary problems

The energy and protein intakes of British 1.5–4.5 year olds is on average adequate to maintain growth, indeed children are taller than they were in 1967/68 when the last major survey of their diets took place. In general, however, preschool children are eating more salt and sugar than is recommended and not enough fruit, vegetables and iron rich foods (see Appendices III and IV). Their diets are therefore inadequate to prevent disease in a number of respects:

- The National Diet and Nutrition Survey (NDNS) for 1.5–4.5 years found that the mean proportion of food energy derived from fat by very young children in the UK is about 36%, but for less advantaged groups it is somewhat higher.
- Consumption of fruit and vegetables is low, although there are no recommended amounts for this age group.
- Average daily intake of iron is below recommended amounts and iron deficiency occurs commonly.
- Intakes of sodium and chloride are above recommended amounts – on average more than twice the Recommended Nutrient Intake (RNI) values.
- Intakes of non–milk extrinsic sugars (sugars such as table sugar, honey, added sugars in processed foods) are too high. For example, children aged 2.5–3.5 are getting almost 20% of total food energy from this source, and some at least a third.
- Consumption of starches and intrinsic and milk sugars is too low. The Committee on Medical Aspects of Food and Nutrition Policy (COMA)

43

Panel on dietary reference values proposed that they should provide on average 39% of total food energy, but they only account for 32%. Some children are only getting 22% of their energy from these sources.

- The children who are receiving nutritional supplements are those who are least likely to need them.[4]

Ethnic and social differences

There are also ethnic differences in feeding practices, with white mothers giving their babies solid food earlier than Asian mothers. By contrast, Asian mothers were more likely to give their baby milk from a bottle longer and their babies had diets with a narrower range than white babies.

In general, the diet of lower socio–economic groups in the UK provides cheap energy from foods such as meat products, full fat milk, fats, sugars, preserves, potatoes, and cereals but has low intakes of vegetables, fruit, and wholemeal bread. In these groups the diet is lower in essential nutrients such as calcium, iron, magnesium, folate, and vitamin C, than that of higher socio–economic groups.

These general characteristics are mirrored in the diets of young children. There is a generally consistent pattern for intakes of total fat and certain fatty acids to be higher for children from less economically advantaged backgrounds, as well as among children whose mothers had no formal educational qualifications.

Children from manual backgrounds:

- Are more likely to eat white bread, and non–wholegrain and low fibre cereals, and buns, cakes and pastries.
- They are only half as likely to drink fruit juice, but are more likely to drink tea.
- They have lower intakes of protein and higher absolute intakes of fat and certain fatty acids (especially monounsaturated fatty acids).
- They have lower intakes of vitamins are recorded for these children and their diets are less nutrient dense, especially in relation to carotene, niacin, vitamin B_{12}, vitamin C, and vitamin E.
- They have lower intakes of most minerals except sodium and chloride. Children of the unemployed had lower mean levels of ferritin ($21 \times g/l$) than children from families where the head of household was economically active ($24 \times g/l$).

There are also differences for family type, with children from lone parent families consuming slightly higher mean energy, starch, fat and fatty acid intakes, but lower intakes of vitamin C and carotene. This suggests that the diets of these children are less nutrient dense. This nutritional disadvantage is exacerbated as the number of children in the lone parent family rises:

children in one parent families with more than one child have lower intakes of calcium, phosphorus and potassium and higher intakes of sodium and chloride than other children do. Children from one parent families with brothers and sisters have the lowest absolute intakes of both carotene and vitamin C.

The children who came from families where the head of household was not working, where the parents were receiving benefits and where the child's mother had no formal educational qualifications, were the most nutritionally disadvantaged.

The health consequences of poor nutrition

One of the foundations of physical and psychological well-being is good food. Receiving a good diet has clear and obvious health outcomes (even if some of them may not manifest themselves for years or even generations to come). Structural and environmental factors, principally inadequate income and inadequate access to healthy food, make it much more difficult for low income families to improve their diets.

Poor nutrition *in utero*

Chapter 8 considers the association between low birthweight and later coronary heart disease (CHD) which is now well established. Fetal undernutrition may lead to a small size and altered body proportions at birth and increased susceptibility to later CHD. The "fetal origins" hypothesis and evidence concerning the role of maternal nutritional status in influencing fetal growth, birthweight and infant and adult disease,[5-7] makes consideration of the high rates of low birthweight in the UK especially important. In addition, life course conditions have a long–term influence on health: nutrition in infancy and childhood may have long–term effects on the initiation of atherosclerosis, and infections acquired in childhood may underlie some of the associations observed.

Figures from the World Health Organisation show that in 1992 the UK had the highest rate of low birthweight babies (less than 2500g) in the EU. At 7% of live births, the UK's rate was on a par with Albania.

Effects on growth

Both the birthweights of babies and the heights of children are lower in deprived areas.[8] An important contributory factor is nutrition. The children of the unemployed, especially the long–term unemployed, tend to be shorter than the children of employed fathers. Unemployment could affect the nutritional status of the under–fours either by lowering the material conditions of the family of the unemployed or by increasing anxiety and depression in members of these families.[9]

Wright et al. compared the heights, weights and head circumference of primary schoolchildren and found evidence of chronic undernutrition among those children from a deprived area. The deprived 5 year olds were on average 2.25 cm shorter than their better–off peers.[10]

Cognitive effects

Inadequate nutrition can impair cognitive development and is associated with educational failure among impoverished children. Recent findings based on a 16 year study of premature babies by the Medical Research Council has provided clear evidence that nutrition early in life has a big impact on the development of the brain. Babies given a "standard" instead of an "enriched" infant formula had significantly reduced language ability and verbal IQ (>85) at 8 years of age (31% of the standard formula group compared to 14% of the enriched formula group). The effect was especially pronounced in boys (47% given the standard formula compared to 13% the enriched formula). Diet during critical periods in early life may therefore be of great importance for our health and performance as adults.[11]

Main nutritional inequality problems and interventions

The key nutritional issues for this age group are breastfeeding, anaemia, dental caries, and obesity.

Breastfeeding

The World Health Organisation stresses the responsibility of every society to ensure that breastfeeding is facilitated in order to encourage the development of each child to its full potential.[12] The documentation of the benefits of breastfeeding is becoming increasingly strong, even in developed countries.[13] James et al. consider that numerous trophic factors, immune cells, polyamines and long chain n–3 fatty acids that are present in breastmilk promote growth and intestinal and brain development. In addition, breastfeeding also avoids inappropriate dietary antigens – from cows' milk and gluten for example – thereby limiting the risk of recurrent infections including diarrhoea, virally induced chest infections, insulin dependent diabetes and atopic disease, until at least adulthood.[14]

Good evidence that nutrition influences cognitive development has arisen from studies of the effect of giving preterm babies breastmilk rather

Table 4.1   Prevalence in UK of breastfeeding at ages up to 9 months: 1990 and 1995

| | Incidence of breastfeeding % | |
	1990	1995
Birth	62	66
1 week	53	56
2 weeks	50	53
6 weeks	39	42
4 months	25	27
6 months	21	21
9 months	11	14

(Source: Department of Health. *Breastfeeding in the UK in 1995*. London: Office of National Statistics, 1997. © Crown Copyright 1999)

than standard formula. The babies given human milk just for 1 month showed major advantages in neurodevelopment at 18 months and in verbal IQ, pattern of allergic reactions and atopy, waist–hip ratio, linear growth, and bone mineralisation at 7.5–8 years.[15] Such effects are biologically plausible, as human milk contains factors including hormones and long chain polyenoic fatty acids that could theoretically influence neurodevelopment. In addition breastfeeding has been associated with a protective effect against insulin dependent diabetes[16] and a reduced incidence of lymphoma.[17] In the UK between 1990 and 1995 there was a statistically significant increase in the incidence of breastfeeding (Table 4.1). The rate for England and Wales increased from 64% in 1990 to 68% in 1995, the increase for Scotland was from 50% to 55% and for Northern Ireland from 36% to 45%. However, although the average rate for initiating breastfeeding in the UK is 66% at birth, it drops 10% in the first week, and by 4 months only 27% of babies are still being breastfed. By contrast in Norway the initial rate of breastfeeding is 95% of mothers.

Inequalities of breastfeeding

Breastfeeding is significantly class related, with women from higher social classes almost twice as likely to choose to breastfeed as women from lower socio–economic groups, with breastmilk providing twice as much energy for infants from the ABC1 socio–economic group compared with those from the C2DE socio–economic group (Table 4.2).[18] Higher rates of breastfeeding are reported among minority ethnic groups. A survey of infant feeding practices among Asian families living in England found that Bangladeshi mothers were most likely to ever breastfeed (90%), followed by Indian (82%), Pakistani (76%) and white mothers (62%).[19] However, among mothers who had ever breastfed, white mothers were more likely to be breastfeeding completely and were also more likely to put the baby to the breast immediately.

Table 4.2   Incidence of breastfeeding by socio–economic group

Socio–economic group	Incidence of breastfeeding %
AB	81
C1	78
C2	65
DE	44

(Source: Mills A, Tyler H. *Food and Nutrient Intakes Of British Infants Aged 6 to 12 Months.* London: HMSO, 1992. © Crown Copyright material is reproduced with the permission of the Controller of Her Majesty's Stationery Office)

Reasons for not breastfeeding are varied

During the first 2 weeks after birth reasons advanced include:

- insufficient milk/baby seemed hungry;
- the mother had painful or engorged breasts;
- baby would not suck/latch on to the breast.

Between 2 weeks and 4 months:

- insufficient milk/baby hungry;
- mother returning to work.[20]

In the UK, if the mother is HIV positive, breastfeeding should not be encouraged as this could increase the risk of transmission of infection and outweigh the benefits of breastfeeding.[21]

Interventions to encourage breastfeeding

In terms of state financial support for breastfeeding, the incentives are the wrong way around. Women on Income Support or from families where the head of household is on Job Seekers Allowance can get free formula, but are not entitled to more money to buy food for themselves if they choose to breastfeed. But the reasons for not breastfeeding or for giving up early are not just economic: complex psychosocial variables, for example social support, maternal maturity, and cognitive ability, may be equally or more important than economic factors in determining infant feeding behaviours.[22]

The link between maternal employment and the early introduction of complementary food has been investigated and confirmed in a number of studies.[23] This suggests that conditions of employment, such as being allowed to take work breaks to breastfeed may be extremely important.

Support for breastfeeding has been largely information based (statements and leaflets announcing that "breast is best") and carried out prenatally with inadequate continuing personal support for mothers who chose to breastfeed.

Table 4.3   Duration of breastfeeding in intervention and control groups in relation to social class (% breastfeeding at each point in time)

	I and II		III		IV and V	
	Intervention (*n*=68)	Control (*n*=83)	Intervention (*n*=120)	Control (*n*=193)	Intervention (*n*=29)	Control (*n*=57)
1 week	99	86	93	89	93	79
2 weeks	96	82	89	83	90	70
4 weeks	84	73	84	74	86	58
3 months	65	55	63	50	45	33
9 months	16	22	15	11	10	14
12 months	6	7	5	5	3	9

(Source: Jones D, West R. Lactation nurse increases duration of breastfeeding. *Archives of Diseases in Childhood* 1985;60:772–4. Reproduced with permission from the BMJ Publishing Group)

There have been few interventions to promote and sustain breastfeeding. Those which have been evaluated demonstrate the importance of continuing social support to maintain breastfeeding rates. Jones and West conducted a randomised controlled trial of a lactation nurse who assisted mothers during the early weeks after parturition both in hospital and home, and showed success in extending the duration of breastfeeding particularly among lower socio–economic classes of women (Table 4.3). By consistent advice and encouragement the nurse enabled mothers to cope more successfully with difficulties and consequently significantly fewer ended breastfeeding prematurely.[24]

Further evidence of the importance of giving close personal support and practical advice in order that breastfeeding may be continued has come from a study at the Institute of Psychiatry and the Children's Department at the Maudsley Hospital. In a small intervention study among 38 working class primiparas between 19 and 32 years,[25] the experimental group was given extra support, viz:

- an immediate visit on their return home from hospital after giving birth;
- telephone contact an available option;
- one or two subsequent visits during the early weeks;
- persistent moral support and practical encouragement.

As the results in Table 4.4 show, there was a significant difference between the experimental group compared to the control group in levels of breastfeeding success.

In trying to identify the exact elements of the intervention which were significant, the author suggests the following:

- the woman was visited in her own home;
- all the consultations were on a one–to–one basis;

- telephone contacts were encouraged;
- continuity in care from pre- to postnatal periods was provided by one person;
- consultation style was non–judgmental, genuine and warm;
- interviewer was informed, experienced and an attentive listener;
- information was given on the supply and demand nature of breastfeeding, on the reasons why breastfed babies cry more than bottlefed ones, and what action to take as a consequence;
- advice was given on the preparation of the breasts prenatally in order to prevent sore and cracked nipples.

However, research in the USA has also shown that successful breastfeeding requires close support during several weeks after birth including help from family and health care personnel, and also societal resources to include workplace opportunities.[22] Research in the USA has shown that the Women, Infants and Children (WIC) program does increase breastfeeding initiation rates.[26] Further research also suggests considerable savings in the USA associated with increasing breastfeeding among low–income women. Taking into account the savings associated with a decrease in infant morbidity, maternal fertility and formula purchases if women breastfed each child for at least 6 months, the authors estimated yearly savings of between $459 and $808 per family. They comment that although many health care providers still view low breastfeeding rates as a cultural choice with no cost for society, this analysis provides evidence that breastfeeding is economically advantageous for individuals and society.[27]

These interventions involved small samples and until they are repeated as a systematic investigation involving a much larger sample and a group of research and field workers, it is difficult to draw firm conclusions. Although the samples in both cases involved working class women, certainly in the Maudsley intervention all the women were arguably more likely to breastfeed because they were keen to breastfeed when pregnant, were neither older nor very young, were healthy and were in permanent partnerships (absence of a partner being a crucial variable). Women from less auspicious backgrounds should be included in further intervention research.

What is needed to encourage breastfeeding?

- Providing personal support for breastfeeding.
- Targeted intervention to focus on the groups most at risk of not starting or not continuing for very long; especially mothers who are young, single, poor smokers, with low educational attainments. These are also the mothers of the babies who probably would most benefit from being breastfed, in that they are more prone to bottle hygiene problems, are passive smokers, and probably had the poorest diet *in utero.*
- Better understanding of the need for continuing support from significant health professionals and family members.
- Local policy guidelines on support of breastfeeding should be published and monitored.
- Help on return to work.
- Greater emphasis should be placed on updating health professionals in order to increase their awareness of breastfeeding issues, promotion, and management.
- Ongoing support for breastfeeding is left largely to the voluntary sector, which is under resourced. Initiatives by lay groups, for example National Childbirth Trust and La Leche League, should be properly subsidised.

Anaemia

Iron deficiency is associated with many biochemical changes and clinical symptoms, with decreased performance, increased susceptibility to infections, and impaired neurological function.[28] The effects of iron deficiency in children under 5 years have been widely reported and include a long–lasting negative effect on growth rate and mental and psychomotor development.[29] Specific groups of the populations in developed countries are at risk. Children from a lower socio–economic background, those fed on cows' milk, and also infants on prolonged breastfeeding have a much higher incidence of iron deficiency than other children. Marx found that in developed countries iron deficiency frequently occurs as a result of low iron intake in underprivileged population groups whose consumption of meat and fresh fruit is restricted by price.[29]

Prevalence of anaemia in the UK

In the UK, anaemia is a significant dietary problem for the 0–5 age group that has been shown to affect all social classes. The National Diet and Nutrition Survey (NDNS) found that one in 12 of all the children in the 1.5–4.5 years age range was anaemic, and in the youngest age group (1.5–2.5 years) this figure was one in eight; it is thought that for Asian children the incidence is more than double (Lawson M, Senior Lecturer in Paediatric Nutrition, Institute of Child Health, personal communication,

51

1997). A comparison of iron intake shows that there has been almost a 22% fall in the amount of iron in the diet in the last 25 years.

Average daily intakes of iron among children aged 1.5–4.5 years are well below the RNI for iron, with 84% of those under 4 years of age and 57% of those aged 4 years and over having intakes below the RNI.

Smaller scale surveys have also shown significant anaemia among poor children. James et al. found that 16% of the children of a general practice in a deprived area in Bristol were iron deficient and 5.8% were anaemic. Among non–Caucasian children the incidence of iron deficiency was much higher – 24% of Afro–Caribbean children were found to be iron deficient.[30]

A recent targeted nutritional intervention programme of 1000 children in areas of high socio–economic deprivation in Birmingham found that 34% of the sample group of children between 18 and 24 months were shown to have haemoglobin levels < 110 g/l. Few of the mothers of children in the sample breastfed their babies beyond 3 months of age and significant numbers of them gave their babies cows' milk before the age of 1 year. The diets of the toddlers were also poor in iron rich foods. Iron deficiency is "the most common nutritional disorder in early childhood" in the UK.[31] Among older children lower iron status is significantly associated with poorer performance in IQ tests and reduced activity levels. (Ash R, Nelson M, unpublished).

Interventions with anaemia

There have been very few intervention programmes in the UK targeted at reducing anaemia (Tedstone A, Lecturer, Centre for Human Nutrition, London School of Hygiene and Tropical Medicine, personal communication, 1997). James et al. showed that health education and counselling when combined with screening can have some success in primary care.[30] The screening programme was offered as part of the routine immunisation against measles, mumps, and rubella.

A more recent study in the UK using health visitors as educators was unsuccessful in reducing anaemia.[31] Combining individual counselling with food vouchers enabling the at–risk population to buy foods containing the essential nutrients deficient in their diets, has been shown to significantly increase haemoglobin levels.[32]

These intervention studies have shown that there are some children who are clinically anaemic who are not currently being detected and treated with iron supplements and dietary advice. Many more will be borderline anaemic. There is no screening programme to detect iron deficient individuals. There is a need for a proper screening and treatment programme targeted at high risk children. Better dietary advice must be given to parents and a greater awareness among teachers and health professionals is needed so that the manifestations of anaemia (under-performance, lack of energy) will not be missed.

Steps can be taken through food fortification to boost iron intake. This has been shown to be important in the WIC programme in the USA through the free provision of fortified formula and foods.[33] Vitamin and especially iron supplementation has also been shown to improve growth status in children aged 3–15 months in Israel.[34]

Excess iron is potentially toxic, can induce tissue damage (for example in atherosclerosis), and is a particular problem for the carriers of genetic haemochromatosis. It would not be appropriate if all parents were routinely encouraged to give their children iron supplements. Intervention cannot be targeted at the general child population but should be directed at high risk communities and individuals. Further research is also required, about the natural history of anaemia in children and what iron levels are important in terms of physical and cognitive outcomes.

Dental caries

Dental caries is a very expensive disease, and there are signs that caries prevalence is now rising in young children in the UK.[35] There is abundant evidence on the dental effects of non–milk extrinsic sugars such as sucrose, with the strongest evidence coming from epidemiology and clinical trials. Caries prevalence is low when fluoride is widely available and consumption of non–milk extrinsic sugars is low. Although fresh fruit is not considered harmful, sugar-containing fruit-flavoured drinks are recognised as being a very great threat to children's teeth. Inadequate tooth brushing is the major determinant of chronic gum disease but is a poor predictor of tooth decay. High levels of dietary sugar are the main cause of tooth decay. While the absolute amount of sugar in the diet is an indicator of the risk of tooth decay, the frequency of its consumption and the way in which it is consumed are often more important predictors. Children who eat sugary foods often and especially between meals, are at the greatest risk of tooth decay.

Water fluoridation is one of the most effective ways of reducing tooth decay in the community – a conclusion supported by the evidence considered by every major independent and government expert committee examining the role of fluoridation of the water supplies.[36] In November 1998, figures published by the National Alliance for Equity in Dental Health (an alliance of 39 national organisations, including the BMA) showed that children in non–fluoridated areas of the UK are up to four times more likely to have teeth extracted due to tooth decay than those in fluoridated areas.[37] It is therefore recommended that all water companies should be legally obliged to ensure adequate fluoride levels in their water supplies, the optimum level being one part fluoride per million parts of water.

Factors associated with dental caries prevalence

The COMA guidelines for consumption of non–milk extrinsic sugars state that they should not provide more than 10% of food energy. At present they provide 17% of children's food energy. The NDNS found that 17% of 1.5–4.5 year old children had some caries experience and in 83% of cases this was untreated. Dental decay is strongly related to social background. The factors most strongly related to caries prevalence are:

* receipt of income benefits in 1.5–2.5 year olds;
* low educational status of the mother in 2.5–3.5 year olds;
* low social class of the head of household in 3.5–4.5 year olds.

Consumption of sugary drinks at bedtime, children being left to brush their own teeth, household expenditure on confectionery and geographical region were also strongly associated with caries prevalence.[38]

Obesity

The prevalence of clinical obesity in Britain has doubled between 1980 and 1991 and is continuing to increase. Obesity exhibits both genetic and familial associations, suggesting an element of individual susceptibility that interacts with adverse environmental conditions to cause extreme weight gain.[39] It is clear that the origins of some adult obesity lie in childhood. Obese children tend to remain obese as adults, but most obese adults were not obese either as children or adolescents. Uncertainty over the precise aetiology of obesity remains one of the chief barriers to designing effective strategies for prevention and treatment.

Overweight and obese adults are at increased risk of morbidity and mortality associated with many acute and chronic medical conditions, including hypertension, dyslipidaemia, coronary heart disease, diabetes mellitus, gallbladder disease, respiratory disease, some types of cancer, gout, and arthritis. The distribution or patterning of body fat in adults is also a risk factor for later disease, independent of the level of obesity.

There are also psychological sequelae: overweight children are more vulnerable to low self–esteem.[40] Indeed, some commentators have noted that the psychological effects of being overweight are more severe than the physiological ones.[41, 42]

Interventions

There is disagreement about whether, and how, to intervene to treat obesity in children. Concern has not only been expressed about the palatability of lower fat diets, but also a child's ability to take in adequate amounts of iron, calcium and calories when consuming lower fat diets. It is especially important that growth is not compromised through provision of inappropriately bulky and low energy diets.[43] The provision of adequate energy and nutrients to ensure growth and development remains the most important consideration in the nutrition of children, and during the preschool and childhood years nutritious food choices should not be eliminated or restricted because of fat content.[44] However, individuals with blood lipids, blood pressure and body mass index in the higher reaches of the distribution in childhood are likely to remain in the upper reaches during adulthood, and a number of processes linked with the development of atherosclerosis may have their origins in childhood.[43]

The most comprehensive and recent literature search[45] argues that population–based approaches to the prevention of obesity are likely to be more effective than approaches targeted at fat children. The Canadian Task Force on the Public Health Examination found insufficient evidence of short- or long–term benefits from screening for, or treatment of, childhood obesity and that most weight reduction programmes have limited long–term effectiveness.[46]

There is a need to focus on activity levels because, certainly among older children, research has shown a trend towards falling levels of physical activity. Active youngsters are less likely to be overweight. Attention and support should also be given to parents of obese children.[40] Activity levels are likely to be linked to fatness even though the evidence is difficult to obtain. Activity strategies become more important at an age when dietary strategies may be of dubious value because they interfere with growth.

The NHS Centre for Reviews and Dissemination recently published a systematic review of interventions in the treatment and prevention of obesity. The review makes the general points that in families where one or both parents are overweight or obese, the children are at greater risk of developing the condition themselves. None of the interventions covered by the report, however, were for the under 5 age group and there were few studies for older children.[47]

What further research is required?

- What influences fatness in childhood and the longer–term impact of childhood environment in later life.
- Effectiveness of interventions, particularly regarding physical activity levels.
- Treatment approaches which enhance the self–esteem of overweight children. A better understanding of the familial and emotional contexts for developing childhood obesity is also required.
- The long–term health impact of fatness originating in childhood.

Inequalities in nutritional status

There are marked differences by socio–economic group in food intake of British infants (see Appendices III and IV). Those from C2DE were less likely to be breastfed (see earlier section in this Chapter) than those from higher socio–economic groups. For the C2DE infants, infant formulas provided 8% of total energy compared to 3% from ABC1 groups. The lower socio–economic infants also had higher energy intakes, obtaining more energy from infant formula, vegetables including potatoes, beverages such as squashes, carbonates and sweetened hot drinks but less from breastmilk and fruit compared with those from ABC1. They also had higher fat, starch, sodium, and total sugars, and less dietary fibre.

Explaining the relationship between nutritional and socio–economic status

Structural and environmental factors, principally inadequate income and inadequate access to healthy food make it much more difficult for low income families to improve their diets and thus their health. The primary determinants of disease are mainly economic and social, and therefore remedies must also be economic and social.[48]

Costs of food

The modern food economy provides a perverse incentive to eat the "wrong" foods because in general the cheapest calories come from fatty, oily foods which are often high in salt and sugar too. It is far cheaper to fill up on a diet of meat products, biscuits, sweets, white bread and margarine than on a healthier diet of fresh fruit and vegetables and lean meat.[49] This "health premium" illustrated in Table 4.5 is, ironically, greater in low income areas.

Shopping access

The geography of food retailing has changed profoundly in recent years, with the food retail market becoming more concentrated in the hands of

Table 4.5   The cost of a basket of healthier food items (wholegrain rice, wholemeal bread, low fat mince, etc.) compared to a basket of similar, less healthy foods

	More healthy basket	Less healthy basket	% Extra cost
Deprived areas	£15.25	£10.84	41%
More affluent areas	£14.87	£11.38	31%

(Source: The Food Commission. *Food Magazine* 1995;**31**(Oct/Dec))

fewer companies. The big supermarket chains now account for 80% of our groceries – 25 years ago it was only 50%. The actual number of shops has dropped considerably too. The Low Income Project Team of the government's Nutrition Task Force found that there has been a general move upmarket as the major retailers have targeted the average and better off, leaving others to aim for the poor. The majority have gained from recent retailing developments, but these have been less than ideal for a significant and growing minority. The effect of the process of polarisation is damaging to the lives and health of people from deprived communities, very costly to the health service and a continuing lost opportunity for Britain's food manufacturing and retailing industries.[50] The collapse of high street shopping and the shift to out of town retailing has been particularly damaging to those without car access.

Piachaud and Webb found that comparing like with like, on average food cost 24% more in small shops such as village shops, corner stores and convenience stores than it did in large shops such as the main supermarkets and discounters. Taking advantage of own brands and "value" products, however, the price difference is much greater: buying the cheapest possible items, as the poor usually do, small shops are 60% more expensive than large ones.[51]

Income adequacy

It is neither lack of knowledge nor lack of thrift that causes some of the inequalities in health, it is lack of an adequate income which denies families the freedom to choose a healthier lifestyle.[52]

In 1995 the National Consumer Council stated in their report *Budgeting for Food on Benefits*[53] that healthy food is beyond the reach of many of the poorest households in the country. The Family Budget Unit has carried out budget studies and compared these figures with Income Support rates to show how far short benefit levels are from achieving acceptable living standards (Table 4.6).

How this shortfall in income is managed by families and its impact on food was the subject of a study funded by the Joseph Rowntree Foundation.[54] They found that four factors appear to determine food choice among low income families:

Table 4.6 Comparison of the low cost budgets and the income support rate for 2 adults/2 child and 1 adult/2 child families: April 1993 prices, £ per week

	Low cost budget	Income support	Shortfall
2 adults/2 children	142.56	108.75	33.81
1 adult/2 children	111.73	88.65	23.08

(Source: Oldfield N, Yu A. *The Cost of a Child*. London: Child Poverty Action Group, 1993)

- However well mothers administered the household budget and tried to ensure that money for food was ring–fenced, in practice this was not always possible.
- Unexpected expenses had to be met and cutting back on food was the only way this could be achieved.
- The problem of reconciling food quality with cost was difficult for parents, but mothers in particular strive to manage their budget and food selection so as to minimise the hardship for their children.
- The cost of food and the money available were the most important factors when deciding what foods to eat.
- In managing the budget, mothers gave priority to the food preferences of other members of the family. Many of the mothers emphasised that they could not afford treats, yet their children received more of their preferred foods, such as chips, beans, burgers, and fish fingers, than their more affluent friends. The reason for this was that the children were being given what they liked in order to avoid waste.

The Family Budget Unit found that state benefits failed to cover the costs of even a budget pared down to a basic minimum. Even without many items which would be deemed necessities by most people, state benefits only covered 74% of this budget for a couple with two young children, and only 77% of the budget for a lone mother with two young children. Evidence shows that when finances are stretched like this food becomes the only flexible item and so bears the brunt of the income shortfall. In 1997 the Family Budget Unit calculated that a couple with two children under 11

Summary of the National Children's Home Poverty and Nutrition Survey (1991)

The difficulty of managing to eat healthily on benefits was demonstrated by the National Children's Home Poverty and Nutrition Survey (1991).[55] In a sample of families attending NCH family centres:

- One in five parents said they had gone hungry in the last month because they did not have enough money to buy food. 44% of the parents said they had gone short of food in the past year in order to ensure other members of the family had enough.
- One in 10 children aged under 5 had gone without food in the last month because they did not like what was on offer and there was no alternative.
- No parent or child was eating a healthy diet. Two–thirds of the children and over half of the parents were eating nutritionally poor diets. Of these, a third of the parents and a quarter of the children were eating very poor diets.
- Poor diet was correlated with food expenditure. The survey showed that there was no evidence to suggest that parents are ignorant about what constitutes a healthy diet. They were unable to provide themselves or their families with an adequate diet because of their income.

would need to spend £79.12 a week on food in order to eat a modest but adequate, healthy diet.[56] In fact families on benefits and low wages spend on average £40.92.[57]

The consequences of inadequate income with which to buy food are most acute when considering the impact on pregnancy. The Maternity Alliance researched the problems faced by pregnant women in affording an adequate healthy diet on present benefit levels. It showed that the cost for an adequate and realistic diet for a pregnant woman would be around £18 a week. However, income support levels – especially for those under the age of 25 – would not support that level of food expenditure. Food would take up nearly 40% of Income Support for single pregnant women over 25, nearly 50% for those aged 18–24, and nearly 65% for single women aged 16–17, an age when they need more nutrients than any other but are eligible for Income Support only during the last 11 weeks of pregnancy.[58]

There have been no interventions in the UK giving people on low incomes extra money and seeing whether they spent it on food, and if so on what foods and with what nutritional effects. A randomised controlled trial in Gary, Indiana has shown that guaranteeing a minimum income to pregnant women in low income families by using negative income tax produced a significant increase in birthweight.[59]

Parental smoking and children's diets

Research in the USA indicates an association between parental smoking and the diet quality of low income children.[60] Children whose parents smoked more than 20 cigarettes a day had a higher level of energy from saturated fat, and children whose parents smoked 11–20 cigarettes a day had the highest cholesterol intakes in comparison with the rest of the sample. In addition, the children of smokers had lower fibre intakes than children of non-smokers.

In the UK, the Policy Studies Institute has also shown that there is a relationship between smoking and diet. Constructing a dietary assessment using a number of food items forgone due to lack of money (a hot meal every day, meat or fish every other day, roast meat joint (or its equivalent) once a week, fresh vegetables, fresh fruit, cakes and biscuits on most days), they compared families with and without smoking parents. In households where both adults smoked, 26% said they could not afford two or more items of food "essentials", in households where no one smoked, 9% said this.[61]

Children and food advertising

Advertising inevitably helps to forge the common culture of acquisition and to fix the parameters of social exclusion in childhood.[62] Children receive a

59

huge amount of attention from food advertisers. Most of the top foods in terms of advertising spend are aimed at children: branded foods in the soft fizzy drink, snack food, confectionery products and sweetened cereals sectors. Food advertising works; there has been an increase in the purchase and consumption of foods which are strongly promoted, and a decrease in poorly promoted foods.[63] In general, there is a marked discrepancy between the foods marketed at children and the nutritional quality of that food, a discrepancy which health professionals or parents may not appreciate.

The trend, at least in homes with cable and satellite TV, is for children to view more television. One recent UK study found that in homes with cable and satellite facilities, children have increased their viewing time by 90 minutes a week between 1992 and 1995.[64]

In the 5 years to 1996 the amount spent on advertising children's food doubled to reach £16 million and it is still growing.[65] Some of this advertising is specifically targeted at younger children – McDonalds has advertisements which are aimed at the under fives and Cadbury's has advertised its "Chocolate for Beginners". Under fives are already brand conscious (Dibb S, Food Commission, personal communication, 1997). Some countries have recognised the vulnerability of young children to advertisers and taken steps to protect them; Australia and Ireland do not permit advertisements during programmes for the under fives.

Poverty and lack of access to affordable alternative leisure facilities probably makes children from low income families exposed to more advertising than children from higher income families. In addition, a way of staying in touch with mainstream culture is through branded goods. Foods like packets of crisps, fizzy drinks, etc. are relatively cheap branded goods and this may also account for their higher consumption among low income households. They are also cheaper ways of keeping in touch with food culture than through eating in a restaurant or a fast food outlet, or buying a take–away. But advertising for branded foods imposes considerable pressures on low income families. Branded foods are more expensive than own–label equivalents, but there is a stigma attached to their purchase and consumption. The Save the Children Charity found that this often means that mothers in such families feel they must buy the expensive branded food – and will even transfer a cheaper version to a branded container if possible, otherwise their children do not want to eat it.[66]

Importance of parental beliefs

The diets of children in this age group are likely to be affected by parents', and particularly mothers', beliefs about food, especially about the importance of healthiness of certain foods. Dowler found that attitudes to food among lone parents in London was significant in accounting for differences in nutritional status among similar income groups. Those who rated ████████████ ariety as important had better diets than those who did not, even if their incomes were similar.

The Head Start nutrition education programme in the USA has shown that a parent education programme can lead to children consuming a significantly more diverse and high quality diet.[67]

Interventions to improve the nutritional status of 0–5 year olds

Interventions should not only be designed to tackle the social and economic reasons that prevent the children of low income families from eating better, but also to increase parents' and carers' beliefs in the importance of choosing healthy foods. Dietary advice that confronts the financial problems faced by parents on low incomes, and stresses practical coping strategies in an acceptable way, is likely to prove most effective.

There are four levels at which nutritional intervention can be aimed: individuals, communities, access, and macro-economic and cultural changes.[68] The vast majority of nutritional interventions have been aimed at individuals. Most nutritional intervention has a behavioural focus and is organised through health workers, such as interventions to improve breastfeeding prevalence. Nutritional education that is mostly aimed at individuals through advice giving has been shown to be ineffective in its present form. It cannot be considered the answer to improving the dietary health of Britain's poor children.

There is a paucity of evaluated interventions that either deal with the major influences on diet – affordability, availability, food beliefs, and skills – or which deal with the specific nutritional problems of this age group. The community based interventions designed to tackle the social, psychological and economic obstacles to low income communities improving their diets need:

• funding;
• properly evaluating for their nutritional and psychosocial impact.

The interventions aimed at dealing with low breastfeeding rates and anaemia:

• have had very small sample sizes;
• have rarely been evaluated;
• have been underfunded.

A mixture of intervention measures are required, but against a background of government commitment to improving the diets and the long- and short–term health of our youngest citizens.

61

Individual interventions

Educating children themselves

Food habits established during the preschool years may affect a person's eating behaviour throughout life, and it is therefore appropriate that good nutritional practices should be taught beginning at the preschool level. Nutrition educators in North Carolina have developed a healthy heart programme for educating children attending day care. It is a 30–40 minute presentation introducing ideas, through the Tin Woodsman character from the Wizard of Oz, about how he plans to take care of his new heart. The programme was used in about 30 day care centres in North Carolina and both preschool children and teachers were said to have responded very positively and enthusiastically to the programme. Parental education to enable them to impart information to their children is also essential.

Peer counselling

There are opportunities to intervene nutritionally by "bolting on" nutritional aspects to other policies. For instance, every local authority has to draw up a policy for education for 4 year olds; nutritional aspects could be written into these policies at a local level. Similarly dietary advice and information could be included in parenting programmes for example Parentlink, Newpin.

Prenatal intervention to increase breastfeeding has been shown to be successful especially when peer group counsellors are employed; that is a woman from a similar racial and socio–economic background who had been a successful nursing mother and who met with the prenatal women during their infant feeding classes to discuss the benefits of breastfeeding.[69]

Community interventions

Providing food in community settings

Low income families who may be least likely to adopt healthy eating habits for themselves or their children, and who may not observe health messages, are sometimes in contact with family centres, for example, National Children's Homes Action for Children Centres. These venues could provide nutritional support and a meals service. For instance the importance of breakfast for ensuring brain function has been noted in several studies of schoolchildren. A number of schools in Britain, particularly in deprived areas, have established breakfast programmes.[70] There have been calls for such programmes to be evaluated to assess whether they are of nutritional benefit to children and whether they have other benefits, such as improving school attendance or reducing disruptive behaviour in the classroom.[71] These programmes and their evaluation should be extended to include nursery settings particularly in deprived areas.

Community based nutritional education

When nutritional education is combined with practical advice, for example what are healthier snacks for toddlers, or even better, accompanied by quasi–cash incentives to purchase healthier foods, then significant nutritional improvement can take place. A good example of this is the Women, Infants and Children (WIC) Program in the USA.

Case study 4.1: WIC program (USA)

Since 1972, the US government has funded the Women, Infants and Children (WIC) Special Supplemental Food Program, the purpose of which is to provide food supplements, nutritional risk assessment, and nutritional education to low income pregnant women, mothers who have recently given birth, and children up to the age of 5.

Reviewing the evaluations made of the WIC program, the General Accounting Office Washington DC found that the most conclusive evidence for success was in the area of infant birthweight. The effect of participation in the WIC program was a 16–20% decline in the low birthweight rate. This effect also applied to the babies of high risk mothers: the babies born to teenage and black mothers participating in the WIC scheme were less likely to be low birthweight and had higher mean birthweights.[72] A more recent meta–analysis shows that providing WIC benefits to pregnant women is estimated to reduce low birthweight rates by 25% and very low birthweight births by 44%.[73]

Improved maternal nutrition through the WIC program has been associated with an increase in infant birthweight, a lower incidence of preterm babies and a longer gestational age.[74]

Participation in the WIC program is also associated with better growth between 6 and 18 months of age.[75] Further research shows that growth rates of infants removed from the program fall back.[76]

In 1990 the WIC program served 4.5 million women and children at a cost of $2.1 billion. The United States Department of Agriculture found that for every dollar spent on the WIC program ensuring low income women an adequate diet during pregnancy, the associated savings in Medicaid costs during the first 60 days after birth ranged from $2.84 to $3.90 for the newborns alone.[77]

The WIC program provided:

- infants up to 12 months of age with iron–fortified formula;
- infants 6–12 months with iron–fortified cereal and vitamin C fortified juice;
- children 1–5 years with milk, adult (iron–fortified) cereal, eggs, vitamin C fortified or citrus juice, cheese, and dried beans.

Lactating women were given milk, cheese, cereal (iron–fortified), eggs, vitamin C fortified or citrus juice, and dried beans.

The WIC program has been particularly successful in reducing iron depletion and iron deficiency anaemia as a number of studies have shown. Infants enrolled in the program from birth have significantly higher ferritin concentration values than infants of similar socio–economic status who were born just before the program started and so were not enrolled.[33] This study showed that fewer WIC infants aged 6–9 months were iron depleted and there was a reduction in the percentage of infants of 9–23 months who developed iron deficiency anaemia.

A meta-analysis of breakfast interventions in the USA, Peru and Jamaica concluded that regardless of research settings, consumption of breakfast consistently benefited the cognitive performance of undernourished children.[78] The conclusions to be drawn from the evidence is that brain function is sensitive to short–term variations in the available nutrient supplies and that the omission of breakfast seems to alter brain function, particularly the speed and accuracy of information retrieval in working memory.

Access interventions

Improved access to food retailing

This includes:

- improving access to low cost food shopping, the encouragement of street markets;
- extending supermarket "value" lines to include more fresh fruit and vegetables;
- improving food distribution on peripheral housing estates;
- making home delivery services available to deprived communities, possibly through a teleshopping terminal at community centres, etc.;
- creating maps of "shopping deserts" and encouraging local authorities and retailers to site new shops in these areas.

Macro–economic interventions

Support with cash: increased resources

Providing low income families with increased resources with which to buy food is likely to improve their nutritional status, but it is not known how much more money would make a nutritionally significant difference. Elaine Kempson calculates that even a modest £15 a week extra can make the difference between "sink or swim".[79] Measures to increase low incomes include:

- statutory minimum wage;
- substantial increases in child benefit, income support, and housing benefit;
- fiscal measures to promote income equality.

With the exception of the first measure, these options do not seem at present to be on the political agenda. However, there are nutritional grounds for arguing strongly that the lone parent premium should be kept and not abolished because children in lone parent families are already at greater nutritional risk. A further drop in their family's income would have serious health consequences.

Support in kind: food, vitamins, and skills training

There are less direct ways of tackling nutritional inequalities, for instance by lifting the burden on poor families' budgets through:

- The provision of a safety net for children at nutritional risk, for example free nursery and school milk, fruit, main meal at minimum nutritional standards.
- Grants not loans for essential cooking items, for example cookers, fridges, home baby food making equipment.
- Teaching cooking skills in school, including eating healthily on a tight budget.

Case study 4.2: Bolton Community Nutritional Assistants Project

The Community Dietetics Service in Bolton and nutrition researchers based at the University of Liverpool have explored the feasibility of using para–professionals or lay persons trained as Community Nutritional Assistants (CNAs) to help identify and address the determinants of dietary behaviour in their local (deprived) neighbourhoods.[80]

Ten people from local communities were recruited and trained. Their task was to explore and act on the food and health needs of local communities particularly in disadvantaged areas, using principles of community development.

The findings:

- After 1 year the CNAs were making four times as many contacts as the community dieticians.
- Flexible working patterns and local knowledge meant they had a unique ability to access typically hard to reach groups: the homeless, hostels, the elderly, the mentally ill, young people, and the unemployed.
- Most contacts involved some form of organised food and health activity such as cook and taste (food skills) sessions or discussions on healthy eating on a limited budget.
- 59% of participants randomly selected for interview said they had made changes in their eating habits as a result of taking part in the project.
- 59% made changes towards buying healthier foods.
- Half claimed they had made changes in cooking practices.

Communicating the message to child care groups

There is a need to disseminate information about nutritional needs of under fives to non–health workers, for example, childminders, nurseries, etc. Chorley and South Ribble NHS Trust has produced Child Nutrition Guidelines to enable parents and carers to be provided with up to date, accurate and consistent advice on feeding the under fives. It has circulated these to nurseries, childminders, the local college for nursery nurse students, and parents (Julie Holt, Health Promotion Dietician, Chorley and South Ribble NHS Trust, written communication, 1997).

Other examples of this include:

- community co–operatives, buying in bulk and distributing to those with restricted access to shops, run without profit;
- community cafes;
- community shops;
- cook and taste sessions;
- recipe books, for instance with ideas for cooking on a tight budget;
- mobile food shops;
- lunch clubs;
- shopping trips in a minibus;
- food voucher schemes.

The National Food Alliance and the Health Education Authority jointly hold a database of these projects. Several of them have children as a specific target.

---

1 Sigman–Grant M, Zimmerman S, Kris–Etherton PM. Dietary approaches for reducing fat intake of pre–school–age children. *Pediatrics* 1993;**91**:955–60

2 Gifft H, Washbon M, Harrison G. *Nutrition, Behaviour and Change*. New Jersey: Prentice–Hall, 1972

3 Gregory JR, Collins DL, Davies PSW, *et al. National Diet and Nutrition Survey: children aged 1 ½ to 4 ½ years*, vol 1. *Report of the diet and nutrition survey*. London: HMSO, 1995

4 Bristow A, Qureshi S, Rona RJ, *et al.* The use of nutritional supplements by 4–12 year olds in England and Scotland. *European Journal of Clinical Nutrition* 1997;**51**:366–9

5 Barker DJ. Fetal and infant origins of adult disease. *British Medical Journal* 1990;**301**:1111

6 Barker DJ, Gluckman PD, Godfrey KM, *et al.* Fetal nutrition and cardiovascular disease in adult life. *Lancet* 1993;**341**:938–41

7 Barker DJ, Meade TW, Fall CH, *et al.* Relation of fetal and infant growth to plasma fibrinogen and factor VII concentrations in adult life. *British Medical Journal* 1992;**304**:148–52

8 Reading R, Raybould S, Jarvis S. Deprivation, low birthweight and children's height: a comparison between rural and urban areas. *British Medical Journal* 1993;**307**:1458–62

9 Rona RJ, Chinn S. Father's unemployment and height of primary school children in Britain. *Annals of Human Biology* 1991;**18**:441–8

10 Wright CM, Aynsley–Green A, Tomlinson P, *et al.* A comparison of height, weight and head circumference of primary schoolchildren living in deprived and non–deprived circumstances. *Early Human Development* 1992;**31**:157–62

11 Lucas A, Morley R, Cole TJ. Randomised trial of early diet in preterm babies and later intelligence quotient. *British Medical Journal* 1998;**317**:1481–7

12 World Health Organisation (1979). In: Jenner S, ed. The influence of additional information, advice and support on the success of breastfeeding in working class primiparas. *Child Care Health and Development* 1988;**14**:319–28

13 Rider E, Samuels R, Wilson K, *et al.* Physical growth, infant feeding, breastfeeding, and general nutrition. *Current Opinion in Pediatrics* 1996;**8**:293–7

14 James WP, Nelson M, Ralph A, *et al.* Socio–economic determinants of health. The contribution of nutrition to inequalities in health. *British Medical Journal* 1997;**314**:1545–9

15 Lucas A. Role of nutritional programming in determining adult morbidity. *Archives of Disease in Childhood* 1994;**71**:288–90

16 Klingensmith GJ. Reduced risk of IDDM among breast–fed children. *Diabetes* 1988;**37**:1625–32

17 Davis MK, Savitz DA, Graubard BI. Infant feeding and childhood cancer. *Lancet* 1988;**ii**:365–8

18 Mills A, Tyler H. *Food and Nutrient Intakes of British Infants Aged 6 to 12 Months*. London: HMSO, 1992

19 Thomas M, Avery V. *Infant Feeding in Asian Families*. London: ONS, 1997

20 Department of Health. *Breastfeeding in the UK in 1995*. London: Office of National Statistics, 1997

21 Royal College of Paediatrics and Child Health. *Recommendations of an Intercollegiate Working Party for Enhancing Voluntary Confidential HIV Testing in Pregnancy. Reducing mother to child transmission of HIV infection in the United Kingdom*. London: RCPCH, 1998

22 Hartley B, O'Connor M. Evaluation of the "Best Start" breastfeeding education programme. *Archives of Pediatrics and Adolescent Medicine* 1996;**150**:868–71

23 Brown K, Dewey K, Allen L. *Complementary Feeding of Young Children in Developing Countries: a review of current scientific knowledge*. Geneva: WHO (unpublished), 1996

24 Jones D, West R. Lactation nurse increases duration of breastfeeding. *Archives of Disease in Childhood* 1985;**60**:772–4

25 Jenner S. The influence of additional information, advice and support on the success of breastfeeding in working class primiparas. *Child Care Health and Development* 1988;**14**:319–28

26 Schwartz JB, Popkin BM, Tognetti J, *et al.* Does WIC participation improve breastfeeding practices? *American Journal of Public Health* 1995;**85**:729–31

27 Tuttle CR, Dewey KG. Potential cost savings for Medi-cal, AFDC, food stamps, and WIC programs associated with increasing breastfeeding among low income among women in California. *Journal of the American Dietetic Association* 1996;**96**:885–90

28 Cook JD, Lynch SR. The liabilities of iron deficiency. *Blood* 1986;**68**:803–9
29 Marx JJM. Iron deficiency in developed countries: prevalence, influence of lifestyle factors and hazards of prevention. *European Journal of Clinical Nutrition* 1997;**51**:491–4
30 James J, Lawson P, Male P, *et al.* Preventing iron deficiency in pre–school children by implementing an educational and screening programme in an inner city practice. *British Medical Journal* 1989;**299**:838–40
31 Childs F, Aukett A, Darbyshire P, *et al.* Dietary education and iron–deficiency anaemia in the inner–city. *Archives of Disease in Childhood* 1997;**76**:144–7
32 Smith AL, Branch G, Henry SE, *et al.* Effectiveness of a nutrition program for mothers and their anaemic children under 5 years of age. *Journal of the American Dietetic Association* 1986;**86**:1039–42
33 Miller V, Sawney S, Deinard A. Impact of the WIC program on the iron status of infants. *Pediatrics* 1985;**75**:100–5
34 Tulchinsky TH, el Ebweini S, Ginsberg GM, Abed Y, *et al.* Growth and nutrition patterns of infants associated with a nutrition education and supplementation programme in Gaza, 1987–92. *Bulletin of the World Health Organisation* 1994;**72**:869–75
35 Rugg–Gunn AJ. Is the concept of non–milk extrinsic sugars valid? *BNF Nutrition Bulletin* 1997;**22**(Spring)
36 Jacobson B, Smith A, Whitehead M. *The Nation's Health: a strategy for the 1990s.* London: King's Fund, 1994
37 National Alliance for Equity in Dental Health. *Inequalities in Dental Health.* November, 1998
38 Moynihan PJ, Holt RD. The national diet and nutrition survey of 1.5 to 5.4 year old children: summary of the findings of the dental survey. *British Dental Journal* 1996;**181**:328–32
39 Prentice AM, Jebb SA. Obesity in Britain: gluttony or sloth? *British Medical Journal* 1995;**311**:437–9
40 Walsh–Pierce J, Wardle J. Cause and effect beliefs and self–esteem of overweight children. *Journal of Child Psychology and Psychiatry* 1997;**38**:645–50
41 Standard A, Wadden T. Psychological aspects of severe obesity. *American Journal of Clinical Nutrition* 1992;**55**:5245–325
42 Weil W. Current controversies in childhood obesity. *Journal of Pediatrics* 1977;**91**:175–87
43 Department of Health. *Committee of Medical Aspects of Food Policy. Nutritional aspects of cardiovascular disease.* London: HMSO, 1994
44 Zlotkin SH. A review of the Canadian "Nutrition recommendations update; dietary fat and children". *Journal of Nutrition* 1996;**126**(4 suppl):1022s–7s
45 Power C, Lake JK, Cole TJ. Measurement and long–term health risks of child and adolescent fatness. *International Journal of Obesity* 1997;**21**:507–26
46 Canadian Task Force on the Periodic Health Examination. 1994 update: obesity in childhood. *Canadian Medical Association Journal* 1994;**150**:871–9
47 Glenny A, O'Meara S. *Systematic Review of Interventions in the Treatment and Prevention of Obesity.* NHS Centre for Review and Dissemination, University of York: York, 1997
48 Rose G. Preventive cardiology: what lies ahead? *Preventive Medicine* 1990;**19**:97–104
49 National Food Alliance. *Myths about Food and Low Income.* London: National Food Alliance, 1997
50 Beaumont J, Leather S, Lang T, *et al. Nutrition Task Force Low Income Project Team. Working Group 2 – policy report.* May 1995 (unpublished)
51 Piachaud D, Webb J. *The Price of Food: missing out on mass consumption. Sticerd Occasional Paper 20. Suntony and Toyota International Centres for Economics and Related Disciplines.* London: School of Economics and Political Science, 1996
52 Stitt S, Grant D. *Poverty: Rowntree revisited.* Aldershot: Avebury, 1993
53 National Consumer Council. *Budgeting for Food on Benefits.* London: NCC, 1994
54 Dobson B, Beardsworth A, Keil T, *et al. Diet, Choice and Poverty.* London: Family Policy Studies Centre, 1994
55 NCH Action for Children. *Poverty and Nutrition Survey.* London: NCH, 1991
56 Parker H. *Modest But Adequate.* London: Family Budget Unit, 1997
57 MAFF. *National Food Survey, 1995.* London: HMSO, 1996
58 Dallison J, Lobstein T. *Poor Expectations.* London: NCH/Maternity Alliance, 1995

59 Smith R. Doctors can reduce the harmful effects of poverty. *British Medical Journal* 1997;**314**:698
60 Johnson RK, Wang MQ, Smith MJ, *et al.* The association between parental smoking and the diet quality of low–income children. *Pediatrics* 1996;**97**:312–17
61 Marsh A, McKay S. *Poor Smokers.* London: Policy Studies Institute, 1994
62 Middleton S, Ashworth K, Walker R. *Family Fortunes.* London: CPAG, 1994
63 Lobstein T. *Myths about Food and Low Income.* London: National Food Alliance, 1997
64 Independent Television Commission. *A Spoonful of Sugar.* London: Consumers International, 1996
65 Register–MEAL/Mintel 1996. *Food Magazine.* 1997;(38):Jan–Mar
66 Save the Children. *Out of the Frying Pan: the true cost of feeding a family on a low income.* London: Save the Children, 1997
67 Koblinsky SA, Guthrie JF, Lynch L. Evaluation of a nutrition education program for Head Start parents. *Journal of Nutrition Education* 1992;**24**:4–13
68 Benzeval M, Judge K, Whitehead M. *Tackling Inequalities in Health.* London: King's Fund, 1995
69 Grossman LK, Harter C, Sachs L, *et al.* The effect of postpartum lactation counselling on the duration of breastfeeding in low–income women. *American Journal of Diseases of Children* 1990;**144**:471–4
70 Harvey J, Passmore S. *School Nutrition Action Groups: a new policy for managing food and nutrition in schools.* Birmingham: Birmingham Health Education Unit, 1994
71 National Dairy Council Nutritional Service. Does breakfast make a difference? *National Dairy Council Quarterly Review* 1996;Autumn
72 Chelimsky E. Evaluations of the special supplemental program for women, infants, and children's (WIC's) effectiveness. *Children and Youth Services Review* 1984;**6**:219–26
73 Avruch S, Cackley AP. Savings achieved by giving WIC benefits to women prenatally (review). *Public Health Reports* 1995;**110**:27–34
74 Brown HC, Watkins K, Hiett AK. The impact of the Women, Infants and Children Food Supplement Programme on birth outcomes. *American Journal of Obstetrics and Gynecology* 1996;**174**:1279–83
75 Heimendinger J, Laird N, Austin J, *et al.* The effects of the WIC program on the growth of infants. *American Journal of Clinical Nutrition* 1984;**40**:1250 7
76 Mora JO, Herrera MG, Sellers S, *et al. Timing of Supplementary Feeding and Its Effects on Physical Growth of Disadvantaged Children.* Boston, MA: Harvard School of Public Health, Nutrition Department, 1981
77 United States Department of Agriculture, Food and Nutrition Service. *The WIC Program.* Washington, DC: Office of Evaluation, 1990
78 Pollitt E. Does breakfast make a difference in school? *Journal of American Dietetic Association* 1995;**95**:1134–9
79 Kempson E. *Life on a Low Income.* London: Joseph Rowntree Foundation, 1996
80 Kennedy L, Ubido J, Price A, *et al. The Community Nutrition Assistant's Project: reorientation or exploitation? 3rd European Interdisciplinary Meeting.* Berlin: Public Health and Nutrition, 1997

Chapter 5 – Childhood injury and abuse

It's like teaching your child to swim in a pool full of alligators.

(Walter Morrison)

Injury and non-accidental abuse of children are a significant source of morbidity and mortality in childhood. Non-accidental abuse casts a long shadow over children's mental and social well-being. The risk of accidental injury is a major cause of anxiety to parents, and poses a restriction on children's freedom.

Child abuse

Child abuse is not the preserve of any one public or voluntary service, and child protection practices are no longer based on the idea that children suffer abuse predominantly because of the unpredictable action of a few disturbed individuals. Much child abuse is not easily detected, and an effective response involves more than the rescue of children, and the conviction and punishment of adults.[1] Professionals from health, social work, education, police and the law are among those with responsibilities in this area, and the differing requirements of, and knowledge bases, attitudes and approach of these organisations mean that well coordinated action, which benefits individual children at risk of, or suffering abuse, and protecting the wider community of children, is fraught with difficulty. The Children Act encouraged a reorientation of services away from an exclusive concentration on detection of cases of suspected abuse and neglect, towards a balance between protection and preventive provision for vulnerable families.

Definitions of child abuse

Four categories of child abuse are defined in the government guidance on child protection for England and Wales. These are:[2]

- *Neglect.* The persistent or severe neglect of a child or the failure to protect a child from exposure of any kind of danger, including cold or starvation, or extreme failure to carry out important aspects of care, resulting in the significant impairment of the child's health or development, including non-organic failure to thrive.
- *Physical injury.* Actual or likely physical injury to a child, or failure to prevent physical injury (or suffering) to a child including deliberate poisoning, suffocation and Munchausen's syndrome by proxy.
- *Sexual abuse.* Actual or likely sexual exploitation of a child or adolescent. The child may be dependent and/or developmentally immature.
- *Emotional abuse.* Actual or likely severe adverse effects on the emotional and behavioural development of a child caused by persistent or severe emotional ill-treatment or rejection. All abuse involves some emotional ill-treatment.

Morbidity and mortality rates of child abuse

Physical, sexual and emotional abuse and neglect

The National Commission of Inquiry into the Prevention of Child Abuse[3] suggests that in terms of neglect, physical and sexual abuse:

- at least 150,000 children annually suffer severe physical punishment;
- up to 100,000 children each year have a potentially harmful sexual experience;
- 350,000–400,000 children live in an environment which is consistently low in warmth and high in criticism;
- 450,000 children are bullied at school at least once a week.

Child injury (abuse)

Child protection registers are sometimes used to provide a proxy for estimates of non-fatal child abuse, but they are generally considered unreliable. The report of children and young people on child protection registers for the year ending 31 March 1998 describes how each social services department holds a central register which lists all the children in their area who are considered to be at risk of abuse and who are therefore the subject of an interagency plan to protect them. It cautions: "the registers are not records of child abuse: some children on the register will not have been the victims of actual abuse; other children who have been victims of abuse will not have been placed on the register if there is no need for a protection plan. These figures should therefore not be interpreted as a record of all child abuse".[4]

There were 31,600 children on the child protection registers at 31 March 1998, representing 28 children per 10,000 population aged under 18. Younger children are more likely to be on the registers than older children. Of the children on the registers at 31 March 1998, 9% were aged under 1, 30% aged 1–4 and 31% aged 5–9. During 1997–98 39% of registrations related to children considered at risk of neglect; this proportion has been rising steadily since 1994. By contrast, the use of the categories physical injury and sexual abuse has fallen.[4] Figure 5.1 details registration during the year ending 31 March 1998, by age, gender and category of abuse. The number of children on a register reached a peak of 45,300 in 1991. Younger children were more likely to be registered than older children.

Registrations and numbers on the register for boys and girls vary widely by age and category of abuse. Of those registered under physical injury during the year, 54% were boys. Girls accounted for 61% of those registered under sexual abuse.[4]

Domestic violence and children

Research provides evidence that domestic violence may begin or escalate in pregnancy.[5,6] Domestic violence can lead to physical and psychological

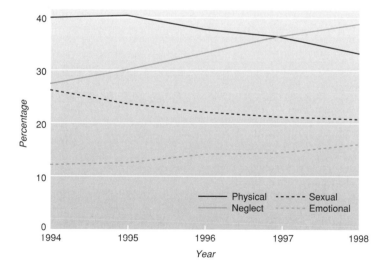

Fig 5.1   Percentage of registrations during the years ending 31 March 1994 to 1998, by category of abuse (including mixed categories). (Source: Department of Health. *Children and Young People on Child Protection Regions. Year ending 31.3.98.* London: HMSO, 1998. © Crown Copyright material is reproduced with the permission of the Controller of Her Majesty's Stationery Office)

harm of the mother and the baby and is associated with adverse pregnancy outcomes such as miscarriage, stillbirth, and preterm labour.[7] Violence within families may continue for many years, and children are affected by violence in a number of direct and indirect ways. Children may be assaulted while trying to stop the violence, being "in the way" when violence occurs, being assaulted as part of the violence to women, or being abused separately. Witnessing domestic violence can cause considerable harm to children in both the short and the long term. In the short term, boys and girls may show a range of disturbed behaviour, including withdrawal, depression, increased aggression, fear, and anxiety.[8] A number of studies have indicated that where there is violence to women in the home, in 40–60% of cases there is also violence to one or more children.[9] In households where there are children, it is estimated that between 75% and 90% of domestic violence incidents are witnessed by the children.[10]

Victims with children fleeing the home may have to live in temporary accommodation or refuges. The Women's Aid Federation England recorded over 50,000 women and children living in refuges in the year 1994–95. Just over 30,000 of those recorded were children.[11] There are a further 52,400 families living in a range of different types of temporary accommodation including bed and breakfast accommodation.[12] Many of these families consist of women and children fleeing domestic violence, others are refugees or asylum seekers. Those seeking refuge or asylum may have gone through periods of extreme violence, including war and the death of friends and family members, or threats to their own and their children's lives, before arriving in Britain.

Child deaths

Children under the age of 1 are more at risk of homicide than any other age group, while children aged between 5 and 15 are the least at risk. In 1992, 38 infants under the age of 1 year were recorded as having died as a result of abuse.

Child injuries

Deaths from injuries remain the greatest cause of childhood mortality and a considerable cause of morbidity.[13] Moreover the gap between the richest and poorest in terms of child injury deaths widened between 1981 and 1991.

Child injury mortality

After the age of 1, accidental injury is the most common cause of death in childhood in the UK. Childrens' injuries result in around 500 deaths a year

73

– a very significantly higher number than those who die through abuse. In 1995, injuries accounted for 4% of deaths among infants aged 1–11 months and 22% among children aged 1–4 years.[14] DiGiuseppi and Roberts analysed unpublished national data for 1992 for children and young people aged up to 19 years, which showed that injury death rates vary substantially by age. The death rate per 100,000 population for all external causes of injuries was 11.7 among children under 1 year of age and 7.4 for ages 1–4 years.[15]

A great majority of child injuries under the age of 5 occur in the home and are most likely to be as a result of burns and scalds, followed by suffocation, drowning and falls and poisoning (Figure 5.2). For children aged 1–4, fire and flames (1.5/100,000) and pedestrian injury (1.3/100,000) showed the highest cause specific death rates. Among children under 1 year of age, the most important cause of injury death was suffocation (2.7/100,000), most of which involved inhalation or ingestion.[15] In England and Wales in 1995 injury and poisoning deaths, both unintentional and intentional, accounted for nearly one in five deaths among children aged 1 month to 15 years (18.5% of the total), and were the leading cause of death among this age group.

Although there has been a fall in death rates from unintentional injury in England and Wales since the 1950s, this has not been as steep as the fall in other causes of death and can be partly explained by changes in travel patterns, especially a reduction in walking and cycling by younger children. In the same period there has been virtually no decline in death rates for intentional injury.[16]

Child injury morbidity

Childhood injuries are a frequent cause of attendance at accident and emergency departments. The most common non-fatal injuries (apart from road traffic accidents) are falls, followed by being struck with an object. Studies in Sheffield and South Glamorgan have shown that in 1 year, one in five of the child population attended hospital because of an injury.[17] A more recent review of these figures found one child in four attending the accident and emergency department in Cardiff in 1 year.[18]

It has been estimated that 2.3 million children attend an accident and emergency department in England and Wales annually. Childhood injuries are also a frequent cause of admission to hospital. Between 5% and 10% of the children who attend hospital are admitted.[19] During the period 1987–89, 19% of 0–4 year olds and 15% of 5–15 year olds consulted their family doctor following an injury.[13]

Data on the long-term consequences of injuries are difficult to access, but one study estimates that about 3% of children under the age of 15 admitted to hospital after an injury have a long-term disability as a result of the injury.[20] Head injuries are the major cause of handicap following injury. Brain damage may also occur following near drowning or suffocation. Burns, scalds and road traffic accidents may result in scarring and cosmetic damage which can be psychologically damaging to the child. The child may be damaged by post-traumatic stress following the accident or from the effects of the subsequent necessary hospital admission and treatment.[19]

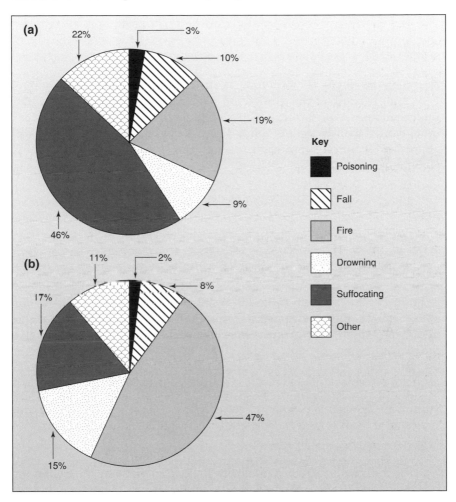

Fig 5.2 Deaths from accidents at home: age and cause, England and Wales 1987–90. (a) Infants 1–4 years: annual mean 109 deaths. (b) Infants under 1 year: annual mean 39 deaths. (Source: OPCS DH4, ICD E850-949, excluding those outside the home. In: Office of Population Censuses and Surveys. *The Health of Our Children: decennial supplement.* Series DS no 11. London: HMSO, 1995. © Crown Copyright 1999)

Health inequalities of injuries and abuse

Inequalities in the exposure of children to risk present a particular challenge to improving the health chances of children. Other European countries – notably the other welfare state countries – have health inequalities, particularly in relation to unintentional injury, which are very much narrower than those in the UK and also lower absolute rates of injury.

Child abuse

Assessing the extent to which there is a social class gradient in child abuse is difficult because of the quality and robustness of data in this area. Our understanding of the factors which contribute to child abuse and neglect is more limited than we care to think. There is not one factor associated with abuse that is not also prevalent among families who do not abuse their children.[21]

The social class gradient

In terms of both child mortality and the social class backgrounds of those who appear on child protection registers, those from the most dis-advantaged backgrounds appear to be at greatest risk. These same families are also, of course, at increased risk of surveillance. Accounts in adult life of those who have suffered abuse in childhood indicate that it is likely that abuse among more advantaged families is underdiagnosed and thus underrepresented. But it seems plausible that there is a real social class difference. Some of this is likely to be related to issues such as overcrowding, where a brief separation between child and angry parent becomes difficult or impossible, and when the effects of poverty can lead to short tempers and anger.

Ethnicity

The needs of black and ethnic minority families are not always well met.[22, 23] Not only is poverty more common among black families and those belonging to certain ethnic minority groups,[24] but also these families include proportionally more young children than white UK families.[25] Research evidence from child protection investigations and interventions confirms that black and ethnic minority families often do not have access to much needed services and suffer additional stress resulting from cultural misunderstandings and language difficulties.[26]

76

Disability

Disabled children may be particularly at risk of abuse. They may find themselves in situations which increase their vulnerability, such as long unaccompanied rides in buses to and from school.[27] They also tend to have a greater number of carers than able-bodied children, be dependent on others for physical and intimate care, and be physically unable to defend themselves. They may be perceived as lacking in credibility if they complain, and disturbed behaviour may be interpreted as the effect of the disability rather than abuse.[28] In terms of disclosing abuse, communicating with a child who has no speech is slow and difficult.[29]

Child injuries

Child injury deaths show the most pronounced social class gradient of any cause of death. The class differences in injury related mortality are greatest for 1–4 year olds, and for boys. Children from poor backgrounds are overwhelmingly more likely than their more advantaged peers to be killed in an accident, and the social class gap has widened over the last decade. Children from social class V have the highest standardised mortality ratios for all types of injuries. Roberts and Power found that the decline in child injury death rates between 1981 and 1991 varied by social class.[30] Information about injuries among minority ethnic children is limited.[31] Those studies which have looked at ethnicity suggest that the influence of poverty is a confounder.[32]

We know less about the social class composition of people who are non-fatally injured than we do about those who die from injuries. However, a number of studies have shown non-fatal injuries to be related to family size (the larger the family the more likely an injury); overcrowded accommodation, housing tenure (injuries are more common in council housing); unemployed fathers, and low levels of parental education. There is an increased injury rate in children of single mothers and young mothers, who are often among the poorest and most isolated groups in the population.[33] The main correlates of child injuries are also indicators of social deprivation.[34, 35] The risk of fire is strongly related to the type of housing, children in temporary accommodation or poor local authority housing are most at risk.[36] The number of families in temporary accommodation has increased fivefold in 10 years.[37] Children living in homes without a play area have five times the risk of being in a pedestrian accident[38] and children living in high rise accommodation are over 50 times more likely to die as a result of falling than are children living on the ground or first floors.[39]

The steep social gradients in child injury risk were quantified over 18 years ago by the Black report, and the inequalities they signalled were targeted as important issues for action and investigation.[40] Yet in the years

77

that have followed, little progress has been made, and indeed, there is some evidence that the gap has widened. Injuries have continued to have a relatively low profile and low priority as a threat to children's well-being.

Effective interventions – child abuse

Although a large investment of professional time and resources has been devoted to the problems presented by parents who provide less than adequate care for their children or who abuse them physically or sexually, studies which robustly assess the effectiveness of interventions in this area are few and far between. Gough's very comprehensive review points out that despite a very high number of publications on child abuse (and on interventions), there is only a relatively small number of formal evaluations. Many of these have serious methodological deficits.[41] More recently, Geraldine Macdonald has assessed the literature.[42]

A number of highly critical public inquiries go some way to explain the preoccupation of professional staff with investigation and monitoring process and procedures in the child protection field, rather than interventions intended to prevent or protect. These factors, together with the variety and combinations of interventions used in research studies, render the task of looking at what works in the field challenging enough, but this is further complicated by:

- variations in the definitions of abuse and neglect used by child care professionals and researchers;
- variations in the conceptualisation of the causes of abuse used in studies (from a failure of attachment, to lack of parenting skills);
- variations in the range, relevance and reliability of outcome measures used, that is, many studies rely on self-reported measures with no external sources of corroboration.

Primary prevention

A systematic review of controlled trials of primary prevention gives pointers on the effectiveness of approaches aimed at reducing the incidence of child abuse and neglect.[43] This review identified 11 prospective controlled trials published in English language journals between January 1979 and May 1993. The interventions studied were as follows:

- Home visits (six studies: two with trained nurses; three with paraprofessionals; one with community mothers).
- Home visits *plus* intensive paediatric contact (one study).
- Enhanced mother–child contact during the postpartum period (two studies one of which compared this with enhanced mother–child contact *plus* home visitation by a paraprofessional).

- Social work following discharge to women regarded at risk for child abuse (one study).
- Early intervention behavioural parent training programme for mother–child pairs identified at risk for child maltreatment (one study).
- Comparison of two programmes, one described as a life-skills, esteem-building programme, the other as a life-skills programme combined with parent training (one study).
- Free transport to appointments for regular prenatal and well-child care (one study).

Not all studies provide adequate descriptions of the *content* of the intervention, for example, what the home visitors *did*, and 11 studies is not many. However, they are among the most rigorous studies in this field, and encompass interventions also evaluated using less stringent designs, so they merit particular consideration. The conclusion reached by MacMillan and her colleagues is that among the perinatal and early childhood intervention programmes, according to the outcomes assessed in their overview, long-term visitation has been shown effective in the prevention of child physical abuse and neglect among families with one or more of single parenthood, poverty, and teenage parent status.[43] The evidence regarding the effectiveness of interventions of short-term home visitation, early and extended postpartum contact, intensive paediatric contact, use of a drop-in centre, classroom education and parent training remains inconclusive.[44, 45]

Child Development Programme

In the UK and Ireland, the Child Development Programme offers monthly support visits to new parents, antenatally and for the first year of life. While not explicitly designed to combat child abuse, the programme nevertheless reports good results in this area. A detailed study of statistical data, across a sample of more than 30,000 programme children in 24 health authorities, trusts and boards, suggests that those families involved in the Child Development Programme have a 41% lower rate of registration on the Child Protection Register, and a 50% lower rate of physical abuse, than adjusted levels for the relevant populations in the same health authorities.[46] The authors caution: "it is necessary to emphasize that the Child Development Programme cannot be used as a kind of anti-child abuse programme. Its success has come about because parents have been supported to become better parents. The programme cannot be used as a selective instrument to target 'vulnerable' parents or those whom professionals consider have a strong chance of becoming abusers. New parents selected for visiting will soon come to recognise that they are being offered the programme because they have been identified as potential abusers, not

79

because they are simply in need of support as parents. When that happens, many parents will simply refuse to have the programme, and rightly so".[46]

Community Mothers Programme

Perhaps the most radical development of this programme is the Community Mothers intervention in which mothers were recruited to provide support. A randomised controlled trial (RCT) demonstrated that children in the intervention group were more likely to receive all of their primary immunisations and to be read to daily. They were less likely to begin drinking cows' milk before 26 weeks. Mothers as well as children in the intervention group had a better diet than the controls. At the end of the study, intervention mothers were less likely to be tired or feel miserable.[47] Since that study was published, the programme has expanded to incorporate breastfeeding support, mother and toddler groups, and attention to the special needs of travellers. In one Dublin suburb a peer led nutrition intervention programme is being developed which draws on the model of the Community Mothers Programme in terms of involving volunteers.[48]

Given reporting biases in child abuse, caution is needed in drawing conclusions about the effectiveness of home visits. However, the Child Development Programme findings, together with the review by MacMillan et al., look promising.[43]

One study was designed in response to suggestions that once child abuse had been predicted, effective prevention was possible.[49] This ambitiously explored the use of data available at birth to predict abuse, and the effectiveness of supportive measures. Eighteen per cent of 2802 non-Asian infants delivered under consultant care in Bradford in 1979 were predicted on the basis of characteristics derived from published studies, and from a local retrospective survey, to be "at risk". Two-thirds of all the recognised abuse in the relevant population occurred in the 18% predicted to be at risk. Those at risk were allocated to a range of social work/health visiting support. The authors report that those who received greatest attention from social workers and health visitors fared worst. While this study raises more questions than it answers, it is difficult to resist the authors' conclusion that although prediction may be possible, the suggestion that prevention is straightforward underestimates the complexity of child abuse.

It is now generally accepted that child abuse, both physical and sexual, and neglect, are the result of a range of variables, biological, psychological, and social. It is important however that we do not lose sight of the influence of macro-social variables such as poverty and inadequate resources. We really do not know the efficacy of tackling portions of the problem of child abuse apart from broader societal needs.[50]

At the personal, familial and community level some of the most promising trends concern interventions derived from learning theories, namely cognitive-behavioural and behavioural approaches, and from systems approaches, in particular systemic family therapy and behavioural family therapy.

Behavioural and cognitive-behavioural interventions

Cognitive-behavioural approaches show promising results in respect of preventive work, and work with families who have injured or seriously neglected their children.

Parent education and training

Parent education or training programmes endeavour to enhance parents' abilities to manage their children's behaviour, to reduce conflict and confrontation while increasing compliance, co-operation and pleasant interaction, and generally to alter the balance of reward and punishment in favour of the former.

While self-reported satisfaction with parenting education programmes is high, the long-term impact, in terms of the increased parenting skills of families impacting on children's social integration and educational performance, as well as on family cohesion, is as yet not fully evaluated.[51] A recent systematic review by Barlow on behavioural changes suggests promising results from well-structured parenting education.[52]

Parent training with families with young children has at its core the following strategies:

- Emphasising the importance of establishing the ground rules and boundaries of acceptable family behaviour, so that children have a growing appreciation of a *plan* against which to assess their own behaviour.
- Helping parents to acquire an understanding of what they can reasonably expect from their children, expecting too much or too little of children of a given age being a common underlying problem.
- Teaching parents to give clear, unambiguous instructions – "James, I want you to . . .".
- Training in contingency management skills – to recognise, reinforce and reward desired behaviour and to acknowledge unwanted behaviour by responding appropriately, for example, ignoring, using non-physical means of punishment such as time-out (a more organised and manageable form of "Go to your bedroom"). Consistency is a key factor.

In general, studies indicate that parent training has good results with a wide range of child behaviour problems, and remains an intervention of choice when skill deficits are identified.[53, 54] It has been successfully deployed by social workers working in the home, in groups, and in family centres.[55]

Long-term follow-up studies with behaviour as an outcome have reported some problems. Some studies record quite high drop-out rates[56] and a failure of successful results to last for any appreciable length of time beyond the end of the intervention or to generalise to new problems.[57] In step-wise fashion, the reasons for these failures have been the subject of investigation, and those factors which appear to be responsible for intervention failures suggest that these are generally attributable to too narrow an approach in response to complex problems. Families for whom parent-training is unlikely to be a *sufficient* response to child management difficulties are those where there is one or more of the following:

- poor parental adjustment, particularly maternal depression;[58, 59]
- maternal stress and low socio-economic status;[60, 61]
- social isolation of mother;[62]
- relationship problems;[63]
- extra-familial conflict;[62]
- the problems are severe and/or longstanding;[64]
- parental misperception of the deviance of their children's behaviour.[56, 65-67]

Two things follow from these data:

- Given the dependence of these programmes on the active participation of at least one parent, this intervention is inapplicable where parents are unwilling to participate.
- The complexity and entrenchment of many of these difficulties indicates the importance of a move away from time-limited approaches with multiproblem families. The development of longer-term therapy has shown dividends in work with families of pre-adolescent antisocial children in contrast with time-limited programmes.[68]

Anger control

Families in which child abuse is a problem are often characterised by low levels of pleasant exchanges and high rates of aggressive behaviour on the part of parent and child. This often results in the all too common "spiralling" in which, in response to a child's misdemeanour, the parents shout; the child continues, they threaten; the child goes on in either the same way or (typically) their behaviour gets worse; parents may smack him, and the child retaliates with verbal and/or physical abuse; the parents "let fly". It is worth noting that the painstaking work of Patterson and his colleagues highlights a problem that bedevils so much research in this area – the predominant focus on mothers and the apparent invisibility of fathers.[68]

Parent-training aims to break this cycle early on by equipping parents with more effective management strategies. However, sometimes the problem lies less with skill deficits of this kind, than in a parent's poor self-control. In most cases, what distinguishes child-abusing families from non-abusing families is not angry feelings or impulses, but that most of the time, the majority of parents can contain these. One of the aims of anger-management strategies is to equip the parent with impulse or anger control – usually in combination with child-management skills.

Training typically involves the following steps:

- The parent learns to identify cues that signal anger. These may be physiological: tension, shaking, "going hot"; or situational: provocative situations such as the supermarket, where the parent feels particularly vulnerable. Some cues overlap both such as tiredness or financial worry.
- The parent learns to relax when these cues are identified and to use various coping strategies. These might include: deep breathing; engaging in an alternative activity; changing the way he or she thinks about the situation.

Helping parents reconstruct their perceptions of situations (cognitive restructuring) often entails providing them with information about age-appropriate expectations of children and here, as with parent-training programmes, there is an overlap with educational approaches.

Choosing alternative courses of action presupposes the ability to think constructively about a situation, to decide what courses of action could be taken, and to choose which would be best. Often, abusing parents are unable to generate alternative (non-aggressive) responses. The resulting stress and frustration contribute to their aggressive outbursts. Like child-management strategies, problem solving can be *taught*, and this has been one component that several self-control training programmes have used.

Because programmes with abusing parents so often include a number of intervention strategies, it is often difficult to say which procedures or which combination of procedures are in fact (the most) effective or responsible for the successful outcomes reported.[69] Whiteman *et al.* compared the effectiveness of four experimental interventions conducted by social workers:[69]

- Cognitive restructuring – aimed at rectifying misattributions of children's behaviour such as "he's doing that to annoy me".

- Problem-solving skills – learning to think of alternative ways of resolving conflicts or dilemmas.
- Relaxation – staying calm so the parent will be less likely to hit out.
- A combination of relaxation, cognitive restructuring, *and* problem-solving skills.

Fifty-five families in which child abuse had occurred, or the parents were at risk for such behaviour, were *randomly assigned* to one of the above four groups and a control group which received agency services but no experimental interventions. The results showed a reduction in aggression measures for those in the experimental groups, with the composite group doing best. While this study relied rather heavily on self-report and role-play measures, rather than on observed real-life situations, their findings are in keeping with a number of other good quality studies conducted by psychologists. There is evidence that groups may enhance the effectiveness or appeal of these approaches.[70, 71]

Family therapy

There are a variety of family therapy approaches. The principles underpinning them suggest that the family is viewed not simply as a collection of individuals but as a rule-governed system and an organised group that transcends the sum of its separate elements.[72]

In viewing families as systems, in which members' behaviour is influenced by that of others, family therapists conceptualise the problems experienced by individual family members as symptomatic of system "malfunctioning". Systems theory recognises that families have to evolve and adapt to the developmental changes of its members (for example, adolescence), changes within the family (children leaving home, death, and so on), and changes outside of it (unemployment, changes in social networks). Family systems are continuously endeavouring both to maintain the status quo and accommodate change (for example, failing to change family rules in recognition of growing children can result in disputes). If they do not manage to strike the balance between the two, problems can occur.

Key therapeutic strategies in systemic family therapy include: *joining* – establishing a bond between the therapist and family members, either singly, or as a whole; *reframing* – a process relationship, or series of interactions, for example helping someone view positively something he or she hitherto viewed negatively; and *prescribing tasks or rituals* – which recognises that much of family life rests on ritualistic patterns of behaviour.

While a number of evaluations of family therapy have appeared in the literature during the last 20 years, statements about its effectiveness as a social intervention in child protection work are particularly problematical for the following reasons;

- There are few studies of acceptable methodological quality.
- While a number of meta-analyses of the effectiveness of family therapy have been conducted, these are problematical insofar as they cover a range of problems (from childhood neurosis to alcoholism for example).
- This problem is exacerbated by the tendency to lump together different family therapy approaches. In a meta-analysis conducted by Hazelrigg *et al.*, only one approach featured in more than one study. This raises the question of whether different family therapy approaches amount to different interventions *per se.*[72]
- Taking mainstream family therapy approaches, we have as yet only slender evidence of the effectiveness of this. This was the conclusion of Hazelrigg *et al.*[72]
- There are too few studies in the literature to reach any definitive conclusions distinguishing between the types of alternative treatments. Before concluding that family therapies are better treatments than other forms of therapy, more and better research must be conducted comparing family therapies with both attention/placebo treatments and viable treatment alternatives.
- Finally, evaluations of family therapy's effectiveness with problems of child abuse and neglect are hard to find, although an exception is described below.

Brunk *et al.* compared the effectiveness of parent training and multi-systemic therapy – systemic family therapy which encompasses attention to the role of cognitive and extrafamilial variables in maintaining problem behaviours, in this case child abuse and neglect. Eighteen abusive and 15 neglectful families were randomly allocated to either parent-training (run in groups) or multisystemic family therapy (conducted in the home). Each programme operated for 1.5 hours over 8 weeks. The authors used both self-report and observational measures (videotapes of parent–child inter-action), and data were collected by research staff who were "blind" to the hypotheses being tested and to the interventions provided to families. The impact of intervention was assessed at three levels: individual functioning, family relations, and stress/social support.[73]

In brief, both parent training and multisystemic therapy appear to bring about statistically significant improvements in the following areas: parental psychiatric symptomatology, overall stress, and the severity of identified problems. Pre-post test comparisons suggested that parent-training was most effective in reducing identified social problems (perhaps because of the group format) and multisystemic family therapy had the edge on restructuring parent–child relationships, and facilitated positive change in

85

those behaviour problems that differentiate maltreating families from non-problem families.[74]

Traditional family therapy approaches are costly given:

- the number of people involved (often up to four per session) and their seniority (though whether this is necessary is a moot point); and
- the high number of "no-shows" and drop-outs from therapy.[75]

Any evaluation of this approach should include an assessment of its cost-effectiveness *vis-à-vis* other approaches.

In terms of budgets and resources, social services departments have tended to give the highest priority to child protection work. In the course of the National Inquiry into Child Abuse, although the question of effectiveness of services was not a central issue, numbers of social workers providing evidence were reported to believe that interventions were effective, and that the most effective intervention was "support".

One means of mobilising support currently being evaluated in the UK is Family Group Conferences.[76] Since the early 1990s, a number of social services departments have been running these meetings, which involve bringing together extended family in the interests of the child, often in difficult circumstances, to discuss child welfare problems, including abuse and neglect. In a study of 80 conferences, 74 produced outcomes which were fully acceptable to professionals and families as being in the best interests of the children and there were indications that children were more likely to have a placement with the extended family, and that the placement is more likely to be stable, following a family group conference.

Discussing *Child Protection: messages from research*, the programme funded by the Department of Health to look at child protection,[21] the Department reminds us that research evidence indicates that around 90% of children have been physically chastised by their families at some point. Summarising a complex area, they write that the evidence suggests that in a generally warm and supportive environment, children who have been hit once or twice seldom suffer long-term effects. But in families who are *low in warmth and high in criticism*, the consequences of negative incidents accumulate, as if to remind the child that he or she is unloved.

One conclusion drawn from a review of child protection research for the Department of Health is that abuse is only one form of adverse childhood experience, and only one aspect of poor parenting. It must not be separated from other areas of individual and interpersonal difficulty.[21, 41]

While the emotional impact of a troubled childhood on both children and their parents cannot be costed, the social costs are clearly vast. Furthermore, the costs disproportionately arise from those who are least well equipped to bear the difficulties and challenges of parenthood. Programmes that increase the power of parents to fulfil their parenting responsibilities – and decrease the likelihood of families experiencing breakdown, delinquency, school exclusion, and abuse – can reduce the need for expensive remedial interventions.[77]

Table 5.1 taken from the National Inquiry suggests a variety of ways in which the range of problems and issues involved might be addressed.

Effective interventions – child injuries

Towner *et al.* reviewed 135 studies and nine reviews evaluating interventions aimed at tackling unintentional injuries on the road, in the home, and in the leisure environment. They showed that the programmes most successful at reducing childhood injury include promotion of bicycle helmets use by legislation or education, promoting the use of child restraint devices and seat belts using legislation, education and loan schemes for home safety improvements, area wide urban safety measures such as traffic calming, and educating children and parents about pedestrian injuries.[78]

Towner *et al.* found few studies that had analysed results by occupational social class. Of those that did, some found that the interventions were less successful among lower social classes whereas others reported success in targeting the lower social classes.[79] For example, Colver *et al.* showed that pre-arranged personal home visits to identify specific targets for change in families living in a deprived area of Newcastle encouraged them to make changes in their homes that would be expected to reduce the risk of childhood injuries. Because there may be a disproportionately low uptake by those at higher risk, it may be important to target such groups with appropriately designed interventions.[80]

Many interventions in children's lives, injury prevention included, are seen as self-evidently a good thing. Preventing children's injuries is frequently done through educational materials. Surprisingly, there is little evidence to support the use of educational materials, and some suggest that it may be hazardous. Ampofo-Boateng and Thomson's[81] review of approaches to child pedestrian injuries in the UK suggests that verbal instructions to children can be hazardous when used in isolation. Behavioural changes advocated by posters and other printed materials are rarely evaluated, and such evidence as there is suggests that changes in knowledge in this area do not readily lead to changes in behaviour. Even when evidence is produced to suggest that health education messages are translated into behaviours, the net result does not seem to be a reduction in risk.[82]

Two before and after studies evaluating the Play it Safe campaign on television found no evidence of reduced hospital admissions, or reduced use of accident and emergency departments.[83, 84] However, education can empower public opinion to institute environmental change. For example,

87

Table 5.1 A child-centred system to prevent harm.

Service	Provider	Aim	Strategy
Information and advice	• Voluntary organisations • Telephone helplines • Statutory agencies • Self-help groups	• Easy access to advice and information on sources of help for: Parents and carers under stress; Children and young people with problems; Members of the public with concerns about the safety of a child	• Central and local government to identify unmet needs for information services and develop plans to meet them • Statutory agencies, including social services, to develop accessible and user-friendly services • Telephone helplines to be effectively monitored and regulated
Child health promotion	• General practitioners • Health visitors • Primary health care team • Hospital staff	• Specified health checks to take account of child protection concerns • Health promotion to include prevention and family support • To follow up *all* children who miss appointments	• Promotion of the core health surveillance programme recommended in *Health for All Children* • Multidisciplinary collaboration between health, social services and education as a response to these checks • Interviews with parents and children to be held in supportive settings, for example, family centres and nurseries
Day care	• Statutory agencies • Voluntary organisations • Community groups and churches • Private sector	• To provide day nursery places to all parents who want them • Day nursery staff to identify children at risk of abuse • Training for nursery staff	• National strategy to be implemented for universal day nursery provision • Maintenance of standards of care across all sectors

Table 5.1   Continued.

Service	Provider	Aim	Strategy
Family support services	• Statutory agencies	• Flexible rate of domiciliary and out-of-home provision to be available to all areas	• Need for family support services to be identified and met through children's services planning mechanism
Education service	• State schools • Independent sector	• All schools to implement child protection guidance and procedures • All schools to develop and implement whole-school behaviour policies • Personal and social education to be provided for all children	• Initial teacher training to include child protection • Headteachers and governing bodies to ensure the child protection system is operating in schools • Inspection bodies to report on operation of systems
Child protection services	• Multi-agency approach: social services/social work, police, health, education	• A swift, non-stigmatising, child supportive response to concerns about child abuse	• To give increased emphasis to family support, while maintaining an effective child protection system • To increase user participation in decision-making
Counselling and treatment services	• Health service • Voluntary agencies • Independent sector • Self-help initiatives	• To ensure that those who have been abused receive counselling and treatment when it is needed	• Area Child Protection Committees (ACPCs)/Child Protection Committees (CPCs) to review provision of treatment services • Central government to issue guidance on provision of treatment • Increased resource allocation

(Source: National Commission on Child Abuse. *Childhood Matters Report of the National Commission of Inquiry into the Prevention of Child Abuse*, vol 1. London: HMSO, 1996. © Crown Copyright material is reproduced with the permission of the Controller of Her Majesty's Stationery Office)

parents can be educated that safe playground equipment is needed for their children. They can then pressure their local authority to act.[19]

A review by Towner et al.[78] for the Health Education Authority looked at the effectiveness of health promotion in the reduction of injuries more broadly, including education, environmental modification and legislation, and the role of healthy alliances. They found no evaluated studies on the use of the law to make drivers more responsible for their actions.

The findings of Towner et al. included the following:

- Broad land use and transport policies, and area wide safety measures have a significant impact on children's use of the environment. They describe a scheme in the Netherlands comparing three packages of safety measures. The first excluded through traffic from residential areas, the second excluded most local traffic, and limited the speed of remaining traffic. The third reconstructed areas as pedestrian priority areas, using the Woonerf model. The second of these proved the most effective, reducing injuries by up to 25%. A UK scheme in five localities to redistribute traffic, and improve the safety of individual roads, resulted in an accident reduction of 13%. The measures which were particularly successful were those which protected two wheeled vehicles at right turns.
- The speed at which a car is driven has a strong relationship to the severity of pedestrian injuries. At 20 mph, 5% are killed.
- There is some evidence that increased wearing of cycle helmets leads to a reduction in injury rates, and fairly strong evidence that it is possible to increase helmet wearing rates by concerted campaigns. However, it is difficult to know whether any fall in injury rates is actually because of a reduction in cyclists on the road rather than reduced risk.
- Product improvements have led to injury reductions, and child resistant packaging of medicine and other hazardous materials has led to a steep reduction in poisonings.

Three observations by Roberts et al.[85] underlie the effective reduction of injuries to children in the context of the family and the community:

- *Most injuries occur in hazardous environments.* Spatial and socio-economic disparities in injury rates are a reflection of differences in the incidence of risky environments. Effective injury prevention is concerned as much with environmental change as with behaviour modification. Road traffic injuries can be "planned out" of particular urban areas through the use of road layout, chicanes, and off street parking. Other injuries can be reduced by attention to housing design, and the provision of safe places for children to play. In practice, between a third and a half of all injuries may be preventable through specific engineering, environmental or legislative measures.[86]

- *Parents and children living in particular environments know a lot about their environments: they are experts in identifying local risks.* At present, much of the data used by those trying to prevent child injuries are insufficiently localised. Moreover, there are no records of child accidents, only of child injuries. These data tend to describe the consequences of an accident rather than the accident itself and its antecedents. Although people living with local risks may become used to them, and even find ways of avoiding them most of the time, on the whole they know what these risks are. The broken fence beside the railway line; the cars that don't stop at the lights even when the green man is showing. Children as young as 7 who took part in a Safe School project[87] were able to identify risks and dangers, and suggest practical measures to alleviate them. Effective injury prevention draws on the specialist local knowledge of children and parents.
- *Strategies among parents for keeping their children safe are more apparent than irresponsible risk taking.* Just as local people are well placed to recognise local risks, they are also likely to have strategies for avoiding these, most of which will be at work most of the time. Prevention policies need to explore the ways in which safety behaviours are integrated into everyday life, and played off against other household routines. (Do I leave my children alone while I go down two floors to hang out my washing, or take them with me down the stone steps?) Effective prevention policies recognise that people living in risky communities are knowledgeable, imaginative and cost conscious and use this expertise.

Family support

An effective way of supporting families with young children which has the potential to reduce injury is through the provision of day care. Day care can provide a safe and stimulating environment for children.[88] Roberts and Pless have also drawn attention to the importance of day care to lone mothers, whose children have injury rates twice those for two parent families – a difference which the authors attribute to poverty and poor housing conditions.[33]

Day care provision is only one aspect of family support, which covers a wide range of services for families bringing up young children in difficult circumstances. Family support services include full or sessional day care, family centres providing direct services as well as advice and counselling, home visiting schemes, short breaks for children with disabilities, and specialist child protection work with families with children on the Child Protection Register.

Social services departments have tended to give the highest priority to child protection work. The results from a major programme of research into its effectiveness initiated by the Department of Health[21] suggested however that this largely reactive work should be complemented by family support

91

services, in order to achieve a more even balance between prevention and protection.[89] Earlier, a 1994 Audit Commission report had recommended increasing the family support provision delivered by family centres combining a wide range of centre based and outreach services.[78, 90]

The introduction in 1995 of mandatory Children's Services Plans which must take account of the links between health, education and social services, gave a further impetus to effective child centred and cross-agency collaboration.[91] These may encourage a more holistic, flexible and comprehensive approach to planning for children's needs, in line with the provisions of the UN Convention on the Rights of the Child.[92] Family support provision offers families the chance to build or strengthen a supportive social network in the community. Good evidence exists for the protective effect on families with young children of community social networks.[93, 94] Family centres in particular provide ample opportunities for children and their parents to meet and make friends.

Although the causes and risk factors of injuries and abuse to children are complex and multidimensional, they are not inevitable outcomes of childhood and can be avoided.

In the UK, no single agency or profession has responsibility for the prevention of unintentional injuries to children, either at national or local levels. Many effective interventions have demonstrated a reduction in injury mortality and morbidity (for example, seatbelt legislation, smoke alarms, traffic speed reduction, etc.), and more needs to be done now to coordinate a national framework for injury prevention that is the responsibility for central government, health authorities, and local authorities. Towner and Ward suggest that this should involve a three pronged attack consisting of legislative approaches, environmental modification, and educational approaches.[95] The importance of multisectoral and synergistic approaches have been demonstrated in this chapter.

1 Directors of Social Work in Scotland. *Child Protection: policy, practice and procedure.* Edinburgh: HMSO, 1992

2 Home Office, Department of Health, Department of Education and Science, Welsh Office. *Working Together under the Children Act, 1989. A guide to arrangements for inter-agency co-operation for the protection of children from abuse.* London: HMSO, 1991

3 National Commission on Child Abuse. *Childhood Matters. Report of the National Commission of Inquiry into the Prevention of Child Abuse.* London: HMSO, 1996

4 Department of Health. *Children and Young People on Child Protection Registers. Year ending 31 March 1998.* London: Government Statistical Service, 1998

5 Hillard PA. Physical abuse in pregnancy. *Obstetrics and Gynaecology* 1985;**66**:185-90

6 Bohn DK. Domestic violence and pregnancy: implications for practice. *Journal of Nurse Midwifery* 1990;**35**:86-98

7 Berenson AB, Wiemann CM, Wilkinson GS, *et al.* Perinatal morbidity associated with violence experienced by pregnant women. *American Journal of Obstetrics and Gynecology* 1994;**170**:1760-9

8 Jaffe P, Wolfe D, Wilson S. *Children and Battered Women.* London: Sage, 1990

9 Hughes HM, Parkinson D, Vargo M. Witnessing spouse abuse and experiencing physical abuse: a "double whammy"? *Journal of Family Violence* 1989;**4**:197-209

10 Hanmer J. Women and policing in Britain. In: Hanmer J, Radford J, Stanko E, eds. *Women, Policing and Male Violence*. London: Routledge, 1989

11 Women's Aid Federation. *Annual Survey of Refuge Groups 1994–95*. London: WAFE, 1996

12 Central Statistical Office. *Social Trends 26*. London: HMSO, 1996

13 Woodroffe C, Glickman M, Barker M, *et al. Children, Teenagers and Health: the key data*. Buckingham: Open University Press, 1993

14 Office for National Statistics. *Mortality Statistics: childhood, infant and perinatal*. Series DH3 no 28. London: The Stationery Office, 1997

15 DiGiuseppi C, Roberts I. Injury mortality among children and teenagers in England and Wales, 1992. *Injury Prevention* 1997;**3**:47–9

16 DiGiuseppi C, Roberts I, Ward H. Childhood injuries: extent of the problem, epidemiological trends and costs. *Injury Prevention* 1998;**4**(suppl):S10–16

17 Sibert JR, Maddocks GB, Brown M. Childhood accidents – an endemic of epidemic proportions. *Archives of Disease in Childhood* 1981;**56**:226–8

18 Mott A, Evans R, Rolfe K, *et al.* Patterns of injuries to children on public playgrounds. *Archives of Disease in Childhood* 1994;**71**:328–30

19 Kemp A, Sibert J. Childhood accidents: epidemiology, trends, and prevention. *Journal of Accident and Emergency Medicine* 1997;**14**:316–20

20 Avery JG, Gibbs B. *Long-term Disability Following Accidents in Childhood. Proceedings of Symposium on Accidents in Childhood*. Occasional Paper 7. London: Child Accident Prevention Trust, 1985

21 Department of Health. *Child Protection: messages from research*. London: HMSO, 1995

22 Caesar G, Parchment M, Berridge D. *Black Perspectives on Children in Need*. Barkingside: Barnardos, 1994

23 Butt J, Mirza K. *Social Care and Black Communities: a review of recent research studies*. London: HMSO, 1996

24 Amin K, Oppenheim C. *Poverty in Black and White: deprivation and ethnic minorities*. London: Child Poverty Action Group in association with the Runnymede Trust, 1992

25 Central Statistical Office. *Social Trends 27*. London: HMSO, 1997

26 Farmer E, Owen M. *Child Protection Practice: private risks and public remedies. Decision making, intervention and outcome in child protection work*. London: HMSO, 1995

27 Westcott H. The abuse of disabled children: a review of the literature. *Child Care, Health and Development* 1991;**17**:243–58

28 NAPSAC. Submission to the National Commission of Enquiry into the Prevention of Child Abuse. *NAPSAC Bulletin* 1995;**11**:10–15

29 Middleton L. *Children First: working with children and disability*. London: Venture Press, 1992

30 Roberts I, Power C. Does the decline in child injury mortality in 1981 and 1991 vary by social class? *British Medical Journal* 1996;**313**:784 6

31 Jarvis S, Towner E, Walsh S. Accidents. In: Botting B, ed. *The Health of Our Children, Decennial Supplement, The Registrar General's Decennial Supplement for England and Wales*. London: HMSO, 1995

32 Alwash R, McCarthy M. Accidents in the home among children under age 5: ethnic differences or social disadvantage? *British Medical Journal* 1988;**296**:1450–3

33 Roberts I, Pless B. Social policy as a cause of childhood accidents: the children of lone mothers. *British Medical Journal* 1995;**311**:925–8

34 Wadsworth M, Burnell I, Butler N. Family type and accidents in pre-school children. *Journal of Epidemiology and Community Health* 1983;**37**:100–4

35 Pless IB, Peckham CS, Power C. Predicting traffic injuries in childhood: a cohort analysis. *Journal of Pediatrics* 1989;**115**:932–8

36 Home Office. *Household Fires in England and Wales: information from the 1994 British Crime Survey*. London: Home Office, 1994

37 Benzeval M, Judge K, Whitehead M. *Tackling Inequalities in Health: an agenda for action*. London: Kings Fund, 1994

38 Mueller BA, Rivara FP, Shyh-Mine L, *et al.* Environmental factors and the risk for childhood pedestrian-motor vehicle collision occurrence. *American Journal of Epidemiology* 1990;**132**:550–60

39 Best R. The housing dimension. In: Benzeval M, Judge K, Whitehead M, eds. *Tackling Inequalities in Health.* London: The King's Fund, 1995

40 Black D, Morris J, Smith C, *et al. Inequalities in Health: report of a research working group.* London: Department of Health and Social Security, 1980

41 Gough D. *Child Abuse Interventions: a review of the research literature.* London: HMSO, 1993

42 Macdonald G. *What Works in Child Protection?* Barkingside: Barnardos, 1999

43 MacMillan HL, MacMillan JH, Offord DR, *et al.* Primary prevention of child physical abuse and neglect: a critical review, part 1. *Journal of Child Psychology and Psychiatry and Allied Professions* 1994;**35**:835–56

44 Hardy JB, Streett R. Family support and parenting education in the home: an effective extension of clinic-based preventive health care services for poor children. *Journal of Pediatrics* 1989;**115**:927–31

45 Olds DL, Henderson Jr CR, Chamberlin R, *et al.* Preventing child abuse and neglect: a randomized trial of nurse home visitation. *Pediatrics* 1986;**78**:65–78

46 Barker WE, Anderson RM, Chalmers C. *Child Protection: the impact of the Child Development Programme. Evaluation Document no 14.* Bristol: Early Childhood Development Unit, Department of Social Work, 1992

47 Johnson Z, Howell F, Molloy B. Community Mothers Programme: randomised controlled trial of non-professional intervention in parenting. *British Medical Journal* 1993;**306**:1449–52

48 Johnson Z, Molloy B. The Community Mothers Programme – empowerment of parents by parents. *Children and Society* 1995;**9**:73–83

49 Lealman GT, Haigh D, Phillips JM, *et al.* Prediction and prevention of child abuse – an empty hope? *Lancet* 1983;**i**(8339):1423–4

50 Garbarino J. Can we measure success in preventing child abuse? Issues in policy, programming and research. *Child Abuse and Neglect* 1986;**10**:143–9

51 Pugh G, De'ath E, Smith C. *Confident Parents, Confident Children: policy and practice in parent education and support.* London: National Children's Bureau, 1994

52 Barlow J. *Parenting Education: a systematic review.* Oxford: University of Oxford, 1996

53 Miller GE, Prinz RJ. Enhancement of social learning family interventions for childhood conduct disorders. *Psychological Bulletin* 1990;**108**:291–307

54 Dumas JE. Treating anti-social behaviour in children: child and family approaches. *Clinical Psychology Review* 1989;**9**:197–222

55 Bourne D. Over-chastisement, child non-compliance and parenting skills: a behavioural intervention by a family centre social worker. *British Journal of Social Work* 1993;**5**:481–500

56 Griest DL, Forehand R, Wells KC, *et al.* An examination between the difference between non-clinic and behaviour problems, clinic referred children and their mothers. *Journal of Abnormal Psychology* 1980;**89**:497–500

57 Griest DL, Forehand R. How can I get any parent training done with all these other problems going on? The role of family variables in child behaviour therapy. *Child and Family Behaviour Therapy* 1982;**4**:73–80

58 Rickard KM, Forehand R, Wells KC, *et al.* Factors in the referral of children for behavioural treatment: a comparison of mothers of clinic-referred deviant, clinic-referred non-deviant and non-clinic children. *Behavioural Research and Therapy* 1980;**19**:201–5

59 McMahon RJ, Wells KC. Conduct disorders. In: Mash EJ, Barkley RA, eds. *Treatment of Childhood Disorders.* New York: Guildford Press, 1989

60 Dumas JE, Wahler RG. Predictors of treatment outcome in parent training: mother insularity and socio-economic disadvantage. *Behavior Assessment* 1983;**5**:301–13

61 Kazdin AE. Premature termination from treatment among children referred for antisocial behaviour. *Journal of Child Psychology and Psychiatry* 1990;**31**:415–25

62 Wahler RG. The insular mother: her problems in parent-child treatment. *Journal of Applied Behaviour Analysis* 1980;**13**:207–19

63 O'Leary KD, Emery RE. Marital discord and child behaviour problems. In: Levine MD, Satz P, eds. *Developmental Variation and Dysfunction.* New York: Academic Press, 1983

64 McAuley R, McAuley P. *Child Behaviour Problems.* London: Macmillan, 1980

65 Lobitz G, Johnson S. Normal versus deviant children. *Journal of Abnormal Child Psychology* 1975;**3**:353–74

66 Larrence DT, Twentyman CT. Maternal attributions and child abuse. *Journal of Abnormal Psychology* 1982;**92**:449–57

67 Reid JB, Kavanagh K, Baldwin DV. Abusive parents' perception of child behaviour problems: an example of parental bias. *Journal of Abnormal Child Psychology* 1987;**15**:457–66

68 Patterson GR, Chamberlain P, Reid JB. A comparative evaluation of a parent training program. *Behaviour Therapy* 1982;**13**:638–50

69 Whiteman M, Fanshel D, Grundy AF. Cognitive-behavioural interventions aimed at anger of parents at risk of child abuse. *Social Work* 1987;Nov–Dec:469–74

70 Nomellini S, Katz RC. Effects of anger control training on abusive parents. *Cognitive Therapy and Research* 1983;**7**:57–68

71 Barth RP, Blythe BJ, Schinke SP, et al. Self control training with maltreating children. *Child Welfare* 1983;**4**:313–24

72 Hazelrigg MD, Cooper HM, Bourduin CM. Evaluating the effectiveness of family therapies: an integrative review and analysis. *Psychological Bulletin* 1987;**101**:428–42

73 Brunk M, Henggeler SW, Whelan JP. Comparison of multisystemic therapy and parent training in the brief treatment of child abuse and neglect. *Journal of Consulting and Clinical Psychology* 1987;**55**:171–8

74 Crittenden PM. Abusing, neglecting, problematic, and adequate dyads: differentiating by patterns of interaction. *Merrill-Palmer Quarterly* 1981;**27**:201–4

75 Howe D. *The Consumer's View of Family Therapy.* Aldershot: Gower, 1989

76 Marsh P, Crow G. *Family Partners: a research study on family group conferences in child welfare.* Sheffield: University of Sheffield, 1997

77 Lloyd E, Hemingway M, Newman T, et al. *Today and Tomorrow: investing in our children.* Barkingside: Barnardos, 1997

78 Towner E, Dowswell T, Simpson G, et al. *Health Promotion In Childhood and Young Adolescence for the Prevention of Unintentional Injuries.* London: Health Education Authority, 1996

79 Downing C. *Evaluation of the Impact and Penetration of a Children's Traffic Club.* Groningen: Second International Conference on Road Safety, 1987

80 Colver AF, Hutchinson PJ, Judson EC. Promoting children's home safety. *British Medical Journal* 1986;**100**:229–35

81 Ampofo-Boateng K, Thomson JA. Child pedestrian accidents: a case for preventative medicine. *Health Education Research* 1989;**5**:265–74

82 Roberts I, Coggan C. Blaming children for child pedestrian injuries. *Social Science and Medicine* 1994;**38**:749–53

83 Williams H, Sibert J. Medicine and the media. *British Medical Journal* 1983;**286**.1893

84 Naidoo J. *Evaluation of the Play it Safe Campaign in Bristol.* London: Child Accident Prevention Trust, 1984

85 Roberts H, Smith S, Bryce C. *Children at Risk? Safety as a social value.* Buckingham: Open University Press, 1995

86 Stone D. *Costs and Benefits of Accident Prevention: a selective review of the literature.* Glasgow: Public Health Research Unit, University of Glasgow, 1993

87 Roberts H. *A Safe School is No Accident.* London: Child Accident Prevention Trust, 1993

88 Roberts I. Family support and the health of children. *Children and Society* 1996;**10**:217–24

89 Cronin N, McGlone F, Millar J. Trends and developments in the UK in 1995. In: Ditch J, Barnes H, Bradshaw J, eds. *Development in National Family Policies in 1995.* York: Social Policy Research Unit, University of York, for the European Commission's European Observatory on National Family Policies, 1996

90 The Audit Commission. *Seen But Not Heard: co-ordinating community child health and social services for children in need.* London: HMSO, 1994

91 Sutton P. All in the same boat – rowing in the same direction? Influences on collaboration over children's services. In: Cohen B, Hagen U, eds. *Children's Services: shaping up for the millennium.* Edinburgh: HMSO and Children in Scotland, 1997

92 Association of Metropolitan Authorities. *Checklist for Children: local authorities and the UN Convention on the Rights of the Child.* London: AMA and Children's Rights Office, 1995
93 Gibbons J. *Family Support and Prevention: studies in local areas.* London: HMSO, 1990
94 Garbarino J, Kostelny K. Child maltreatment as a community problem. *Child Abuse and Neglect* 1992;**16**:2455–64
95 Towner E, Ward H. Prevention of injuries to children and young people: the way ahead for the UK. *Injury Prevention* 1998;4(suppl):S17–S25

Chapter 6 – Physical, sensory and cognitive disability

Truly a handicapped child is a handicapped family . . . it is society which imposes the greatest burden on parents and carers.

(E Younghusband, 1974)

Definitions of disability

The WHO definition discusses "disability" under three key headings, namely:

- *Impairments*: any loss or abnormality of physiological, psychological or anatomical function or structure (for example, paraplegia), medically definable conditions, or diseases (for example, cystic fibrosis).
- *Disabilities*: any restriction or loss arising from an impairment, of the ability to carry out an activity in a way or within the range that would be considered normal for a person of a similar age (for example, the inability to walk).
- *Handicaps*: the impact of the impairment or disability upon the individual's pursuit or achievement of the goals which he/she wishes or expects, or which are expected by society (for example, the inability to read or to walk, which may prevent independent living or employment).[1]

However, the WHO terminology has in recent years aroused considerable anger among the growing number of organisations for disabled people. Coleridge[2] has argued powerfully for a social rather than a medical model of disability, with a recognition that it is not the disability but the negative attitudes of society which "handicap" disabled people. In 1991, Disabled Peoples International adopted a definition of disability (strongly supported by the British Council of Disabled People) which states that:

> Disability is the loss or limitation of the ability to take part in the normal life of the community on an equal level with others, due to physical and social barriers.

Hutchison[3] notes the importance of having definitions which are positive but which enable services to be accurately targeted and which do not inadvertently disadvantage some disabled people by failing to specify unmet health or other needs.

Hall[4] notes that children's disabilities can usefully be separated into three broad groups, namely:

- High severity, low prevalence conditions: these conditions will usually have a substantial and permanent impact upon a child's quality of life and future development. Such conditions include blindness, severe learning disabilities, sensorineural deafness and severe cerebral palsy.
- Developmental or neurodevelopmental conditions or disabilities: learning disability, emotional and behavioural problems, speech and communication disorders and a range of difficulties such as speech delay, reading difficulties or clumsiness, which do not necessarily fit into neat diagnostic categories.
- Low severity, high prevalence conditions: include more minor conditions or disabilities which are probably of organic origin, but do not usually have a profound impact on the child's future. These may include conductive hearing loss; squint; myopia.

Prevalence and patterns of disability

It is estimated that there are 327,000 children with disabilities in the UK under the age of 16.[5] The Office of Population Censuses and Surveys (OPCS) includes children with emotional and behavioural difficulties in its definition of disability and the study notes that many children's disabilities will not be identified until they enter school. The Inner London Education Authority[6] estimated that 68% of pupils with disabilities, special educational needs or emotional and behavioural problems, were unidentified until entering the school system. The high incidence of undetected disabilities or special needs reflects in most cases social disadvantage; lack of family mobility and no previous contact with relevant professionals. In considering definitions of disability, it is also important to recognise that disability is seldom a single condition. Parker[7] reanalysing OPCS data for the Department of Health, has concluded that the average number of disabilities experienced by disabled children under the age of 5 living at home was 2.6, rising to 9.6 for children with the most severe disabilities. The most commonly reported disability was behavioural, with up to 80% of children in residential care being identified as having behaviour difficulties.

For some children, the severity of the primary disability may be less "disabling" to everyday life than a secondary disability (such as a behavioural problem) which impedes quality of life.

A list of the major diagnoses of chronic disability is given in the box below.

Risk factors of disability

Low birthweight and special needs

Kemply et al.[8] in a study in South London noted that the relative risk that very low birthweight infants would have subsequent special educational needs amounted to a risk of 4.4 times more than normal birthweight infants, and that these findings mirrored an earlier Finnish study. However, they stress that the increased risk for special educational needs may be the result of social as well as biological factors in this group of children.[9–11] O'Callaghan similarly notes the connection between increasing survival of very low birthweight infants and subsequent educational and other disabilities. The study provides detailed educational outcomes on a range of academic measures and shows significant educational difficulties in many of the children (46% requiring remedial help and 4% attending special educational provision). However the study notes that the families' social, ethnic and educational backgrounds might influence the level of the child's

---

- Speech and language impairments (including developmental and acquired dysphasia, etc.). The incidence depends upon definition but it is estimated that there are at least two severe and persistent cases per 1000 births.
- Severe learning disability (mental handicap): 3.7 per 1000 births.
- Epilepsy is estimated to affect 50 000 children in the UK: 15% of children affected have additional learning disabilities and cognitive disabilities.
- Hearing impairments: the Royal National Institute for the Deaf estimates 64 000 children have a significant hearing impairment in the UK.
- Visual impairment: the Royal National Institute for the Blind estimates that there are 20 000 children with significant visual impairment in the UK, with 60% having additional learning or physical disabilities.
- Diabetes is increasing in children across Europe: 1 in 1800 children aged 0–9 are estimated to be affected.
- Duchenne Muscular Dystrophy: 3 per 1000 male births.
- Cerebral palsy: 1.5–3 per 1000 births.

difficulties and access to early intervention and support, and stresses the importance of early intervention to assist the children educationally and limit the social consequences of later school failure.[9]

Pharoah and Cook[12] looked at the association between very low birthweight and the subsequent incidence of cerebral palsy, and concluded that among infants weighing 2500 g or less, not only was there a tenfold risk increase over that for normal weight babies, but there was also a significantly higher risk in multiple than in singleton births. An increased risk of disability and mortality in twins is significant because of the growth of multiple births, largely as a consequence of infertility treatment. However as Botting[13] comments from the Office of National Statistics, there is an urgent need for reliable data on the incidence of cerebral palsy in the UK and for the long-term follow-up of multiple birth babies.

Learning disabilities

There is an estimated prevalence of severe learning disability of 3.7 per 1000 children. Learning disability may have multiple causes, including specific syndromes (in particular Down's syndrome or fragile X); associations with other disabilities such as cerebral palsy or epilepsy; or postnatal insults such as meningitis or trauma.

It had been anticipated that the incidence of syndromes like Down's syndrome would be considerably reduced because of selective abortion following improved antenatal screening techniques. However, as Hall[4] notes, the incidence of one in 660 births has remained constant for Down's syndrome over a number of years. Although the risk of Down's syndrome is linked to maternal age, the majority of women have their babies in their twenties or early thirties. Overall, the prevalence of this condition is not significantly reduced by screening programmes targeting older mothers.

Hearing and visual impairments may have an impact upon a child's development and subsequent educational opportunities. Conductive hearing loss is extremely common and at least half of all preschool children will have one or more episodes of otitis media with effusion (OME). The extent of disability caused by OME is still controversial, but severe and persistent OME may result in significant delay in language acquisition; behaviour difficulties, and in some cases temporary balance problems. Hall[4] and Haggard[14] note that hearing loss interrelates with other factors such as environmental deprivation (which in turn may delay diagnosis).

Visual impairments are also important in the early years. Hall[4] identifies four key reasons for early detection:

• Some conditions are treatable (for example, cataracts or glaucoma).
• Many visual impairments have genetic implications.

- Developmental guidance and early educational advice is highly valued by parents (and probably reduces the incidence of secondary disabilities such as behaviour problems).
- Social deprivation may also affect early identification because of families' inability to use services or because the child does not attend any service where screening takes place.

Speech and language problems can cause major concerns to parents and to preschool services. There is some evidence that very slow development of language may be caused by socio-economic factors.[4] However the connection is not strong and it is important to avoid seeing delayed language development as an isolated phenomenon. It will often be accompanied by other problems which can include autism or learning disabilities, hearing impairment or cerebral palsy. Importantly, impaired language development of whatever origin may interrelate with other factors such as developmental delay, behavioural problems and adverse social circumstances to severely affect the child's general growth and development. Appropriate early identification may in effect break the spiral.

The inequalities of disability

For disabled children born into socially disadvantaged families, multiple disadvantages, such as poor housing, parental unemployment, lack of family or community support, homelessness or parental ill health may all have a powerful impact upon parental coping strategies. A report from the University of Bristol states there are approximately 150,000 families caring for severely disabled children in Britain who slip through the net in terms of meeting their housing needs. The research shows that poor or unsuitable housing has a significant impact both on the care burden imposed on parents and, equally importantly, on the degree to which a disabled child can attain as independent and normal a childhood as possible.[15]

The financial inequalities of disability

An important and well documented feature in the lives of many families with a young disabled child is that of the cost of disability and the associated social as well as economic consequences which result from the additional financial burden on families.[5, 16–22]

Surveys from the OPCS have found that families with a disabled child, regardless of social class, were substantially worse off than families with able-bodied children. OPCS found that 73% of fathers of disabled children were in full time employment, as compared to 88% of the general population of fathers.[23] Baldwin,[24] also using Family Fund data, found that

33% of mothers of young disabled children, as compared to 59% of mothers in the general population, were working and that if they did work they tended to work shorter hours and for below average pay. However, OPCS[5, 20, 21] found that a high proportion of mothers of disabled children wished to work – not only for financial reasons but because employment offered social status and friendship. In a review of the literature on social support for disabled children and their families, Baldwin and Carlisle concluded that disability in a child both creates a need for additional expenditure and at the same time reduces the income available to pay for this by restricting the labour force participation of both mother and father.[25]

Both Baldwin and OPCS note the special and additional difficulties encountered by single parents with disabled children. OPCS found 30% of single parents (as compared to 17% of couples) were in financial difficulties. Not surprisingly these families were also more likely to say that their health was affected by having a disabled child and that their inability to work was in part related to the absence of a supportive partner.

Many families caring for a disabled child face additional costs such as additional heating, the purchase of aids and equipment (for example, incontinence aids and medicines, wheelchairs and mobility aids), the replacement of furniture and household equipment, and transport costs. Loughran et al.[22] found that notwithstanding their greater need, families with disabled children were less likely to have telephones; to be able to purchase new clothing or household equipment or to own a car than other families with non-disabled children. Parker[7] concludes that using this data, 55% of households with a disabled child were living in poverty or on its margins in 1985. These households had (and probably still have) a greater likelihood of living in poverty than any other social group including lone parents or families with disabled adults.

Parker notes that it is not clear how far the poverty of this group of families was precipitated by a disabled child or how far poverty and social inequality were exacerbated by the impact of disability. However, this analysis has important consequences both for social policy towards families and for the development of more effective child health promotion policies within disadvantaged communities.[7]

Parker demonstrates that among families with disabled children, the lowest 20% of income received fewer services than all other families. For example, 16% of families with incomes in the top three income bands used special furniture or custom-made equipment. This fell to 4% in the lowest income band. Similarly 20% of children with identified locomotion difficulties (in families within the top three income bands) had mobility aids, whereas numbers plummeted to 4% in the poorest fifth of families.[7]

Beresford[26] found when analysing Family Fund data that families with the most severely disabled children often demonstrated the highest number of unmet needs. Single parents and families from minority ethnic groups were particularly at risk. Baldwin[24] found that even basic living costs were increased by having a disabled child in the family. The difference would amount to £20 per week increased expenditure in middle income families, if adapted to 1996 prices.

Russell[27] in a survey of parents' views in a London authority found that shortfalls in family budgets limited effected use of available services. Low income families were particularly likely to raise the issue of transport costs, one mother observing that she frequently missed appointments made for her child because the travel costs on unreliable and inconvenient public transport were simply too high.

Parker noted that foster families usually received a good level of support when caring for a disabled child. Their access to improved levels of services could be simply explained by the existence of explicit local authority policies to support vulnerable children "looked after by the local authority" and, in most instances, the availability of good information, professional support, respite care and other services as part of a "package of care". Some natural parents have argued that if such resources were targeted at families with disabled children prior to family breakdown, then that investment might well prevent expensive family placements and enable natural families to continue caring.[7]

Ethnic minority families

A particularly disadvantaged group of families with disabled children in all studies[1, 22, 26, 28] are those from minority ethnic groups. Beresford found families from minority ethnic groups were among the most disadvantaged in the survey.[26] The barrier of inadequate information and lack of interpreters, the reluctance to offer some services such as respite care because of misunderstandings about the role of the extended family and the poor housing and poverty exacerbate any problems of care.[29]

Emerson[28] in a study of Asian carers in North West England, found that 65% of families had difficulties in paying basic bills when there was a disabled child in the family. Only a minority could speak (37%) or write (24%) English and hence had little knowledge of services which might have supported them. On a formal measure of health-related stress, four out of every five carers reported levels of stress which indicated a real risk of developing mental health problems in the future. Over 40% of mothers reported back problems, chest pains, depression, and weeping. Notwithstanding the high levels of physical and social deprivation, all families wished to care for their children at home. The barriers were primarily those of maintaining a reasonable quality of life and sufficient income to meet the family's needs.

Targeting resources is often ineffective and significant numbers of the most disadvantaged families (that is, families where disability, low income and social disadvantage create multiple jeopardy) are the least likely to get support. The Disability Living Allowance (DLA) is often not applied for because parents are not aware of it and the qualifying criteria.[30] Health care professionals need to be more aware of this and promote a greater uptake of the allowance. This in turn could reduce financial burdens and inequity.

Abuse in disabled children

An American study[31] found that disabled children were 17% more likely to be sexually abused than non-disabled children. They were twice as likely to be emotionally neglected or physically abused. This study also suggested that some impairments might actually be caused by abuse – an estimated number of 147 disabled children in a sample of 1000 abused children. A Canadian study estimated a 50% increased risk to disabled children, with evidence that multiple disability or severe levels of disability increased the risk still further.[32]

In the UK a small snapshot study by the NSPCC of referrals of disabled children found 84 disabled children, 34 of whom had physical and/or learning disabilities. The largest group of perpetrators were peers (that is, other children) or staff. Seventy-one per cent of the children had been abused by more than one perpetrator and 26% of the perpetrators had previous histories of child abuse; 39% of the allegations of abuse resulted in criminal prosecutions.[33] Kennedy[34] carried out a major survey of abuse on deaf children and found 192 suspected cases of abuse and 86 confirmed cases of physical and emotional abuse, with 70 cases of suspected sexual abuse and 50 confirmed cases. She concluded that not only were disabled children more vulnerable to abuse, but also if abused, they were likely to experience abuse for longer periods than other children without disabilities.

Westcott[35] identified some key factors which predispose disabled children to abuse, namely:

- Physical and social isolation.
- Multiple caregivers – the Council for Disabled Children found some disabled children had 40-50 different carers (including transport). These carers were likely to be managed through multiple agencies. Some were provided through agencies on a block contract basis, with few details known about their past.[36]
- Lack of choice (parents may feel pressured to use a service they feel is inadequate because they cannot manage without support).
- Lack of physical and psychological resources for self-protection; disabled children may have limited communication skills; may be heavily dependent on others for personal care, and may have such limited life experiences that they have difficulty in interpreting inappropriate behaviour.

104

- Physical immobility (that is, the child may be unable to get away).
- A desire for affection and attention (which may make the child vulnerable).
- Pressures of care (which may make family or professional carers impatient, careless, or sometimes punitive in care regimes).
- A lack of belief that anyone would want to abuse a disabled child.
- A perception that disabled children cannot be regarded as sound witnesses and therefore prosecution is unlikely, even if the abuse is detected.

Since the publication of the Younghusband report[37] in 1974, there has been an ongoing debate about the optimum models for the early identification, assessment and application of appropriate interventions for preventing abuse for young children with disabilities and their families. The same decades have seen growing awareness both of the importance of listening to and empowering parents as key educators of their own children and of the need to ensure that families have the social, family and financial support that they need to carry out what are often very challenging tasks.

The debate about early identification and intervention has to be put in the wider context of social change in the UK over the same period. There are increasing anxieties about polarisation of resources between the socially disadvantaged and their more affluent peers. The concept of "social exclusion" has received much attention at government and local level. An agenda for action on "excellence for all" in education has highlighted the importance of actively involving parents in their children's development. But there is corresponding awareness that many parents will need considerable support in order to play such a role and that wide variations and fragmentation in services can make empowerment and participation very difficult.

The shift in population of children with impairments towards more severe and complex disorders, a greater ethnic and cultural mix in Britain than before, and a greater proportion of single parents and families living in poverty have changed the patterns of needs to be addressed without a parallel shift in professional aims, attitudes and practice (despite forward looking legislation like the Children Act 1989).[38]

Notwithstanding concerns about fragmentation of services and growing evidence of social deprivation, there have been positive changes in services for disabled children and their families. There is growing interest in evidence based interventions, for ongoing monitoring and evaluation of different models of care and support, with parental satisfaction seen as an important measure of effectiveness, and also for child-centred measures.[39, 40] There is also growing awareness of the need for parent support, advice, and advocacy.[41, 42] Most importantly, parents of disabled children themselves are becoming more articulate, actively involved in the development and sometimes the direct management of local services and are frequently involved in individual programmes to encourage their child's development.[43]

Offering comprehensive, coordinated and effective assessment, advice, information and relevant support for children with disabilities and special needs and their families will always be challenging. Early identification and diagnosis (whether in education, child health, or social services) will always be fraught with ethical and practical difficulties. Social disadvantage and deprivation may delay identification in some cases because of family mobility or inability to access services. Poverty and its associated consequences of poor housing, social isolation, unemployment and parental ill health, may limit parents' abilities to engage in programmes with their child or even to attend services. A growing minority ethnic population presents new challenges with regards to information, accessibility and understanding of cultural and linguistic needs which, if ignored, will also constitute barriers to services.

The early years present particular challenges in developing flexible and effective services for young children with disabilities and their families and although children's abilities and needs may change over time, their disability will be life long.[38] However, the child's functional impairments may not be reliably predictable at an early stage. Parents and professionals will in effect need to find an appropriate balance between treatment and other interventions (with their implications of "labelling" and possible "cures") and on the other hand helping parents to enjoy and value their child as a child first and a disabled person second.

Parents may blame themselves if they cannot "cure" their child's disability or be under considerable pressure from family and community to try new and alternative approaches. Conversely adverse social circumstances may turn a child's relatively modest impairment into a significant handicap, which isolates him or her from ordinary activities in family and community.

Meeting the needs of young disabled children and their families has to be seen as a collective responsibility. Services as far as possible need to be local, flexible and move beyond the traditional model of identification, assessment, treatment and review. In this context child health services may need to act as advocates to local housing departments to improve families' living environments; to ensure that families receive all the benefits to which they are entitled to combat poverty, to maximise children's participation in educational activities, and to provide a family policy which enhances the family's ability to cope.

Attitudes and expectations have changed. The management of early identification, diagnosis and assessment of disability in the early years has greatly improved. But many families are still seriously disadvantaged[7, 26] and unless their social circumstances are addressed, other interventions will be ineffective or underutilised.

Family policy support

The past decade has seen an unparalleled interest in (and accompanying debate around) the role, rights and responsibilities of families. The debate has in part been positive. Most policies are moving away from "crisis intervention" towards refocusing around family support and "early intervention". But at the same time there is growing uncertainty within a contract culture about what style of early intervention can actually help children and families and at the same time represent value for money. Equally, there has been an emerging intolerance towards difficult and disruptive children; about parental responsibilities and rights and an increasingly punitive attitude towards those children who do not fit in easily within the current framework of services.

In the UK (as in many other countries), the UN Convention on the Rights of the Child has stimulated new interest in children's rights and family policy. It also provides a framework for early identification and intervention, in particular identifying key themes which need to run through any policy developments. These four themes are:

- Participation: the concept of the child as an emergent and active citizen.
- Provision: to be made on the basis of a child's right to health, education, and care.
- Protection: acknowledging the right of all children to be safe and protected from abuse.
- Community: the right to a family life, friendships and inclusion in the local community.

Most countries are seeing major competition between resources for children's services and the needs of an increasingly large and frail elderly population. The Audit Commission[44] and others have emphasised the importance of more targeted investment in vulnerable children and families and the need to see prevention as being a critical issue in promoting the "well-being" of children. However, any discussion of how best to target families in order to promote the well-being of children necessitates an understanding of family lifestyle and structures and, in particular, how such lifestyles and structures may be affected by disability and disadvantage.

Dale[42] examines a range of models for developing a framework for understanding the family (with a disabled child). She groups these models into three main categories, namely:

- The Pathological or "Sick Family" Model assumes that families are disabled by having a disabled child. Family problems are because of the "abnormal" child.

107

- The "Common Needs" Model describes "ordinary families" with exceptional needs.
- The "Stress and Coping" Model describes families with disabled children as having the capacity for a rich and varied life, but with ordinary life experiences interspersed with periods of considerable stress.[42, 45, 46]

In the UK the assumption is that children's needs cannot be met by a single professional but that the professional with the "hands-on" responsibility must be able to implement a range of interventions and work with a multi-agency team to resolve any problems.

There is a network of Child Development Centres associated with paediatric departments which have evolved over the last 30 years. They provide a multidisciplinary assessment and therapeutic intervention pro-grammes. These should continue to be linked to tertiary care paediatric neurology departments to ensure accurate diagnosis. The outcome of the child is dependent on establishing a full profile of the child's problems and developing a co-ordinated plan to meet them.

There is an increasing range of early intervention programmes which involve families in a variety of educational activities. Portage is the best known and evaluated in this country and has been highly effective in developing parental confidence and competence in helping their child to develop. Like High Scope, Portage can also offer flexible packages to disadvantaged families and offers a home-based service.

Dale[42] suggests the development of key indicators for intervention. She hypothesises that it is possible to identify the characteristics of families who are most likely to experience stress and to invest in these families. Key factors appear to be:

- Reluctance to accept a diagnosis or a disability.
- Reporting of behaviour problems (particularly sleep disturbance).
- Multiple disabilities.
- The mother is socially isolated, without a network of family or friends, and with low self-esteem.
- Financial difficulties.
- Lack of family cohesiveness and mutual support and respect.
- Passivity rather than positive utilisation of existing support or suggested coping strategies.
- Lack of strong moral or religious beliefs.
- Poor housing.

An important characteristic of a number of recent innovative approaches to developing parent-friendly services has been asking families what they want. A survey by Family Fund Trust[47] asked parents to prioritise the services they needed to care for a disabled child at home. All parents were caring for severely disabled children and met the Family Fund Trust criteria for support. Priorities were similar across all age groups, with help with holidays, family outings and leisure activities a high priority. Practical help with equipment, home safety and laundry followed rapidly. But the emphasis upon holidays and leisure also reflects the importance of such activities for family life – and for a sense of family well-being at a time when many local authorities are significantly reducing budgets for holidays and leisure activities.

Developing a policy of children and family support

Currently we have little evidence of the long-term outcomes of different styles of family support (as opposed to outcomes for educational interventions). The Mental Health Foundation,[48] in a report of a Committee's Inquiry into children with learning disabilities and challenging behaviours, highlights the urgent need to prioritise evaluation and research into the different models currently available and notes the importance of such an approach at a time when evidence based treatments or interventions are the preferred options for many purchasers. However outcome measures may be different when measured against the family's increased self-confidence, the child's improved behaviour or educational development, or society's satisfaction that a "problem" has been solved.

Since 1996, local authorities have been required to produce Children's Services Plans, which should provide interagency strategic planning for children in need within all local authorities. The planning requirement has highlighted the challenge of producing accurate and relevant information on local populations of disabled children.

Baldwin and Carlisle[25] reviewing the research literature on services for disabled children concluded that support systems for all families caring for a disabled child need to ensure:

- The availability of accurate and accessible information for parents, professionals and purchasers of services after identification of disability.
- A recognition of the emotional and social context of assessment and utilisation of services and any special provision.
- An acknowledgement of the stress under which some parents live on a day-to-day basis – the treble jeopardy of stress, disadvantage and disability.
- Active support for parents, whose personal circumstances make it difficult to use parent networks and other community support systems for information, advice, and practical help.
- A commitment to the principle of maximum inclusion in good quality children's services.
- A recognition that some children have very complex needs.

Short-term breaks

Short-term breaks (which may vary from day care only through to several weeks or longer in family crises) is universally highly regarded by parents. However, there is growing evidence[19, 29] that families with the greatest need may not receive a respite care service because of pressure on waiting lists and lack of information about accessing services. Aldgate,[49] examining the wider implications of short-term breaks for families with children who would be regarded as being "in need" as well as having disabilities, concludes that short-term care needs to be considered as a range of models, namely:

- Breaks are highly valued by families. Contrary to some fears that short-term breaks may "teach a family that life is easier without a child", parents also value the time available for other family members and often form friendships with their children's carers, and children enjoy short-term breaks and the relaxation and play opportunities they provide.
- Preparation for parents and children is crucial. Some disadvantaged parents may regard short-term breaks as "taking children into care" unless reassured. Carers in turn need to be willing to commit time and concern to working with natural parents and accepting their anxiety.
- Family support services should be available before the first crisis. They can be particularly helpful when poverty, isolation and lack of support feature among family problems. Some vulnerable parents have lacked positive "mothering" experiences themselves and the right respite care service may compensate for this lack.

Early identification

Early identification and intervention are not only issues for child health services, although education and social services are likely to heavily depend upon the role of child health services in identifying potential need and vulnerability in children under 5. Conversely, programmes like Portage[50] clearly demonstrate that families can be the most effective and economical system for fostering and sustaining the development of a young child through working with families and can enhance parental ability to utilise health as well as other services more effectively.

As the UN Convention on the Rights of the Child tells us, the family is the fundamental group in society and the natural environment for the growth and well-being of all its members. But important questions remain about the most effective and acceptable models of early identification and intervention and how we move away from the concept of "parents as problems" to a more pro-active partnership approach which acknowledges strengths, weaknesses and aspirations within a constantly changing society. It is certainly clear that in addressing issues of inequality and disability, it is essential to adopt a multifaceted approach to both the context and the content of any early identification or intervention programmes. As Hall[4] notes, the aims of child health promotion programmes are:

- to promote "good enough parenting";
- to reduce the incidence of developmental, emotional and behavioural disorders, parental depression and distress and child abuse and neglect (primary prevention);
- when prevention is not feasible, to identify any disorder or disability as early as possible (secondary prevention);
- to provide support and care for children with permanent disabilities and their families (tertiary prevention).

For disadvantaged families, the interrelationship between primary, secondary and tertiary prevention and the promotion of "good enough parenting" will be critical. "Parent education" is currently much under discussion, though not necessarily well understood.

The past decade has seen a major growth in early intervention and support programmes for young children with a range of different special needs and their families. As the Mental Health Foundation[48] notes, evidence of long-term effectiveness is seldom available and there is an urgent need for more systematic monitoring and evaluation of different programmes. However, notwithstanding variable degrees of monitoring and evaluation, there are some well developed programmes.

Homestart

One example is Homestart, founded in 1973, which provides regular support, friendship and practical help at home to families with young children who are under pressure. Although not formally evaluated, the befriending role for disadvantaged families has been widely endorsed. Homestart is not specifically concerned with disability, but it can support vulnerable families with children with a range of special needs and parents in accessing a wider range of services.

Newpin

Newpin (New Parent Infant Network) provides a package of social involvement, therapy and training through 10 centres in England. Centres offer creches and drop-in facilities, but the key to the programme is the matching of mothers with a trained volunteer befriender. Early evaluation demonstrates primary benefits for mothers through an increase in self-esteem and parenting skills.

111

Portage

Portage is the best known of the home teaching programmes. It is a programme for parents and children with disabilities or special educational needs within the UK, but originated in the USA as an educational tool for disadvantaged parents, to encourage active participation in their child's development. The strength of Portage has been its ability to develop parents' skills as early educators of their child; to provide access to a range of professionals through the home teacher; and to target intervention at areas of concern for parents as well as professionals.

High Scope

One of the best evaluated early intervention programmes is the USA High Scope compensatory education programme. High Scope[51, 52] offers high quality "compensatory" education for the children of poor mothers. While one of the project's original aims of increasing children's IQ has not been proven, the scheme's long-term evaluation has demonstrated that it has longer-term important achievements, in particular[48] improved performance at school and in the employment market place, reductions in teenage pregnancy, substance abuse and offending, and greater stability in children's adult relationships. The association with reduction in offending has interested the Home Office in the UK, which is currently investing in a number of pilot schemes.

Parent advisers

Some early intervention programmes have been specifically targeted at parents of young disabled children. Cunningham and Davis[41] and Dale[42] describe the role of the parent adviser – a trained professional or volunteer who works with parents of young disabled children to encourage active participation in their child's development and to increase confidence and competence in helping their child. In one locality, health visitor and paediatric clinical medical officers were trained in a specific model of parent counselling, including work on parenting and child behavioural management. Under the supervision of a clinical psychologist, they provided a direct service to families in the catchment area for two health centres in Lewisham and Southwark. Benefits found included improved self-esteem and reduction of stress in the mothers, improvements in the home environment, and decreased behavioural problems in children. The parents also had lower consultation rates with primary health care staff. The service was provided under the auspices of the Lewisham and Guy's Mental Health Trust.

The evaluation of the parent adviser scheme (initiated in the London Borough of Tower Hamlets) found that the service had the greatest impact on the most disadvantaged families (particularly those from the local Bangladeshi community for whom same-background parent advisers were generally identified).

Larner *et al.* stated that the past decade has seen growing interest in early intervention and family support for families with young disabled children (in particular those from socially disadvantaged backgrounds). However with broader definitions of intervention, the concept of "early intervention" for identified disabilities or special needs such as family disadvantage may have different objectives for different agencies. The evidence for effective intervention may be directed to: specific cognitive goals; the prevention of later offending; parent education; protecting vulnerable children from harm; or ensuring that early education or other programmes are initiated right from the start for disabled children.[53]

The management of disability in early childhood is challenging. The Children Act 1989, in introducing a concept of "children in need" and including children with disabilities within mainstream children's legislation, set a new agenda for interagency support for disabled children and their families. In practice, management of the initial diagnosis and assessment remains complex, with many parents still feeling frightened, marginalised, and insufficiently informed. Parents clearly value an integrated approach to diagnosis, assessment and intervention, and there is encouraging evidence of much creative work by child development centres and teams, often in conjunction with local social services and educational initiatives.

Research from Beresford[26] and others confirms that families with the greatest needs may actually receive the fewest services. Less articulate, more isolated and often with pressing social problems, they will need advocacy and support in order to make best use of available services. Data from the Family Fund Trust,[47] OPCS[5] and Parker[7] clearly demonstrate the additional costs of disability and the real hardships experienced by many families with disabled children.

Disadvantage and inequality need not accompany disability if there are robust local planning arrangements which ensure easy access to disability specific services, and also take account of the social, demographic, ethnic and economic composition of the local community. The "well-being" of young disabled children and their families will only be achieved if we can create active partnerships which see children and families as key players in their own futures and acknowledge the mutual and important responsibilities of all statutory services.

John is not a handicap, he is not a syndrome, he is not a problem, he is my son. The first thing we parents want from doctors, all those professionals out there, is the recognition that a child has been born. We usually celebrate birth – but not if we have a disabled child! We parents of disabled children are often treated as problems, a convenient free treatment resource. But we are still a family. The UN Convention said it all – that we should work together towards

113

"the development of the child's personality, talents, and abilities to the fullest potential in conjunction with the development of respect for the child's parents, cultural identity and values". What do we want from the health service? We want advocacy, commitment, respect. Above all else understand the day-to-day problems that we parents live with and recognise that it is society and inequality which create the handicaps of living with a child with disability, not the disability itself. (Parent speaking at European seminar on early intervention. Quoted In: Carpenter B. *Families in Context: emerging trends in family support and early intervention.* London: David Fulton Publishers, 1997)

1 World Health Organisation. *International Classification of Impairments, Disabilities and Handicaps.* Geneva: WHO, 1996
2 Coleridge T. *Disability, Liberation and Development.* Oxford: Oxfam (UK and Ireland), 1993
3 Hutchison T. *Definitions of Disability: towards a nationally useful definition, Report of Working Party.* Bath: British Association of Community Child Health, 1996
4 Hall D. *Health for All Children,* 3rd edn. Oxford: Oxford University Press, 1996
5 Office of Population Censuses and Surveys. *The Prevalence of Disability Amongst Children. OPCS surveys of disability in Great Britain, Report 3.* London: HMSO, 1989
6 Inner London Education Authority. *Equal Opportunities for All? Report of Committee of Inquiry to review special educational needs in the Inner London Education Authority.* London: ILEA, 1996
7 Parker R. Counting with care; a re-analysis of the OPCS data. In: Social Services Inspectorate and Council for Disabled Children. *Disabled Children; directions for their future care.* Wetherby: Social Services Inspectorate/Department of Health Publications, 1998
8 Kemply S, Diffley F, Ruiz G, *et al.* Birthweight and special educational needs: effects of an increase in the survival of very low birthweight infants in London. *Journal of Epidemiology and Community Health* 1995;**49**:33–7
9 O'Callaghan MJ. School performance of ELBW birthweight children: a controlled study. *Developmental Medicine and Child Neurology* 1996:**38**:917–26
10 La Pine TR, Jackson J, Bennett F. Outcome of infants weighing less than 800 grammes at birth. 15 years experiences. *Pediatrics* 1995;**96**:479–82
11 Johnson A, Townsend P, Yudkin P, *et al.* Functional abilities at 4 years of children born before 29 weeks gestation. *British Medical Journal* 1993;**306**:1715–18
12 Pharoah P, Cooke T. Cerebral palsy and multiple births. *Archives of Disease in Childhood* 1996;**75**:174–7
13 Botting B. Cerebral palsy and multiple births. *Archives of Disease in Childhood* 1996;**75**:174–8
14 Haggard M. Hearing and screening in children – the state of the art(s). *Archives of Disease in Childhood* 1990;**65**:1193–5
15 Oldman C, Beresford B. *Homes Unfit for Children; housing, disabled children and their families.* London: Joseph Rowntree Foundation/The Policy Press, 1998
16 Glendinning C. *Unshared Care: families with disabled children.* London: Routledge and Kegan Paul, 1983
17 Beresford B. Resources and strategies; how parents cope with the care of a disabled child. *Journal of Child Psychology and Psychiatry* 1994;**35**:171–211
18 Russell P. *The Role of the Named Person.* London: Council for Disabled Children, 1996
19 Russell P. *Positive Choices: services for disabled children living away from home.* London: National Children's Bureau, 1996
20 Office of Population Censuses and Surveys. *Mortality Statistics: perinatal and infant; social and biological factors.* Series DH3/25. London: HMSO, 1993
21 Office of Population Censuses and Surveys. *The OPCS Monitoring Scheme for Congenital Malformations.* Occasional Paper 43. London: HMSO, 1995

22 Loughran F, Parker R, Gordon D. *Children with Disabilities in Communal Establishments: a further analysis and interpretation of the Office of Population Censuses and Surveys' Investigation. Report to the Department of Health, from the Department of Social Policy and Social Planning.* Bristol: University of Bristol, 1992

23 Bradshaw J. *The Family Fund: an initiative in social policy.* London: Routledge, 1980

24 Baldwin S. *The Costs of Caring: families with disabled children.* London: Routledge, 1985

25 Baldwin S, Carlisle J. *Social Support for Disabled Children and their Families: a review of the literature.* Edinburgh: HMSO, 1994

26 Beresford B. *Expert Opinions: families with severely disabled children.* York: Policy Press/ Joseph Rowntree Foundation, 1995

27 Russell P. Parents as partners: some early impressions of the implementation of the code of practice. In: Wolfendale S, ed. *Working with Parents of SEN Children after the Code of Practice.* London: David Fulton Publishers, 1997

28 Emerson E, Azmi A. *Improving Services for Asian People with Learning Disabilities and their Families.* Manchester: Hester Adrian Research Centre, 1997

29 Shah R. *The Silent Minority: children with disabilities in Asian families,* 2nd edn. London: National Children's Bureau, 1996

30 Steadman P. The new Disability Living Allowance. *Archives of Disease in Childhood* 1993;**68**:73–4

31 Crosse S, Kaye E, Ratnofsky A. *A Report on the Maltreatment of Children with Disabilities.* Washington DC: National Center on Child Abuse and Neglect, 1993

32 Sobsey D, Varnhagen C. *Sexual Abuse and Exploitation of People with Disabilities.* 1988 (unpublished thesis)

33 National Society for the Prevention of Cruelty to Children. *Childhood Matters: the report of the national inquiry into the prevention of child abuse.* London: NSPCC, 1996

34 Kennedy M. The deaf child who is sexually abused – is there a need for a dual specialist? *Child Abuse Review* 1990;**4**(2):3–6

35 Westcott H. *Experience of Child Abuse in Residential Care and Educational Placements: results of a survey.* London: NSPCC, 1993

36 Council for Disabled Children. *Children with Disabilities and Special Needs: current issues and concerns for child protection procedures.* London: Council for Disabled Children, 1997

37 Younghusband E. *Living with Handicap. Report of a Committee Inquiry.* London: National Children's Bureau, 1974

38 Ball M. *Disabled Children: directions for their future care.* London: Council for Disabled Children and Social Services Inspectorate, Department of Health Publications, 1998

39 Appleton P, Boll E, Kelly A. Beyond child development centres, care coordination for children with disabilities. *Child Care Health and Development* 1997;**23**(1):29–41

40 King G, Rosenbaum P, King S. Evaluating family-centred service using a measure of parents' perceptions. *Child Care Health and Development* 1997;**23**(1):47–63

41 Cunningham C, Davis H. *Working with Parents: frameworks for collaboration.* Milton Keynes: Open University Press, 1985

42 Dale N. *Working with Families of Children with Special Needs: partnership and practice.* London: Routledge, 1996

43 Cameron R. Early intervention for young children with development delay: the Portage approach. *Child Care Health and Development* 1997;**23**(1):11–29

44 Audit Commission. *Seen But Not Heard: co-ordinating child health and social services for children in need.* London: HMSO, 1994

45 Davis H, Buchan L, Choudhury P. Supporting families of children with chronic illness and disability. In: Mittler P, Mittler H, eds. *Innovations in Family Support for People with Learning Disabilities.* Lancashire: Lisieux Hall Publications, 1994

46 Davis H. *Counselling Parents of Children with Chronic Illness or Disability.* Leicester: British Psychological Society, 1993

47 Family Fund Trust. *What Would be of Most Help to You in Caring for Your Disabled Child?* York: Family Fund Trust, 1995

48 Mental Health Foundation. *Don't Forget Us: children with learning disabilities and severe challenging behaviour. Report of Committee.* London: Mental Health Foundation, 1997

49 Aldgate J. *Children In Need.* London: HMSO, 1995

50 Cameron R. A problem-centred approach to family problems. In: Daly B, ed. *Portage: the importance of parents.* London: NFER/Nelson, 1983

51 Schweinhart LJ, Weikhard DP. *A Summary of Significant Benefits: the High-Scope Perry pre-school study through age 27.* Michigan: High Scope Press, 1993

52 Home Office. *Preventing Children Offending: a consultation document.* London: Home Office, 1997

53 Larner M, Halpern R, Harkavy O. *Fair Start for Children: lessons learned from seven demonstration projects.* New Haven: Yale University Press, 1992

Chapter 7 – Emotional and behavioural problems

Childhood is not just a preparation for life, it is a part of life . . .

(Anon.)

There has been a rise in the rates of various psychiatric disorders in young people since the Second World War.[1] These disorders frequently begin in childhood[2] and are often a source of considerable distress to the children involved, their families, or both. The current challenge is to develop and implement effective primary and secondary preventive initiatives on a widespread and equitable basis, in the context of co-ordinated strategies to meet the health, developmental and educational needs of early years children.

Definitions of mental health

Children's mental health is not simply the absence of mental ill health, but can be described in its own right. The NHS Health Advisory Service review of child and adolescent mental health services uses the following definition:

The components of mental health include the following capacities:

- The ability to develop psychologically, emotionally, intellectually and spiritually.
- The ability to initiate, develop and sustain mutually satisfying personal relationships.
- The ability to become aware of others and to empathise with them.
- The ability to use psychological distress as a developmental process so that it does not hinder or impair further development.[3]

117

Within this broad framework, and incorporating the developmental nature of both body and mind in childhood and adolescence, mental health in young people is indicated more specifically by:

- A capacity to enter into and sustain mutually satisfying relationships.
- Continuing progression of psychological development.
- An ability to play and learn so that attainments are appropriate for age and intellectual level.
- A developing moral sense of right and wrong.

This definition is intended to describe the mental health of children in general. Mental health in infants needs special consideration, because it is intimately connected with the capacity of the primary caregivers to appreciate, interpret and manage their child's emotional and physical needs. Where the relationship between a young child and the caregiver is "good enough",[4] this has a beneficial effect on many aspects of the child's development. In particular, children are more likely to develop secure attachments, a positive sense of self, and an accurate awareness of their own and others' emotions. These attributes are important foundations for mental health.

Mental health in infants and young children, while strongly influenced by the capacity of parents to provide adequate care, also needs to be understood in a wider context. There is a complex interrelationship between the child's genetically determined characteristics, the family's competencies and problems, the support and services available in the wider community, the quality of the physical environment, and the degree to which government policy is family friendly.

From this broad perspective, it is apparent that a variety of agencies, both statutory and non-statutory, will have an impact on the mental health of young children. This needs to be acknowledged in planning initiatives promoting young children's mental health.

Many children will experience an impairment in their mental health at some point. For these children, the nature of their problems may be conceptualised in different ways. Leaving aside the variety of intrafamilial and cultural explanations which may be evoked for their difficulties, health services, education services and social services will often think about these children using different language and emphasising different aspects of their problems. These differences can breed misunderstanding and inhibit communication. For example, psychiatrists tend to distinguish between normal and abnormal groups of children, and think of the abnormal group as having disorders with specific characteristics, treatments, and outcomes. They see these disorders as produced by an interaction of biology and environment. Teachers, and others involved in education tend to use an undifferentiated category of "emotional and behavioural problems". They see these as primarily caused by adverse environmental factors, in particular problems in the family context, and perceive them as essentially amenable to improvement through education. Social workers and workers in the voluntary sector tend to regard labelling children as a stigmatising process which is best avoided, and prefer to explain children's problems in social terms. These descriptions are of course stereotypes, and there will be many exceptions to the characterisations presented. For example, many GPs and health visitors often think more like teachers and social workers than typical medical professionals. But the problem of different languages and conceptual frameworks in different professional groups is a real one. It inhibits the multidisciplinary collaboration which is so important across and within the different services involved with young children: the NHS, social services, education, and the voluntary sector.

The Health Advisory Service[3] distinguishes three levels of severity in children with impaired mental health:

- Mental health problems: relatively minor conditions such as sleep disorders or excessive temper tantrums.
- Psychiatric disorder: marked deviation from normality together with impaired personal functioning or development and significant suffering.
- Mental illness: severe forms of psychiatric disorder, particularly of the kind also found in adulthood, for example, schizophrenia, depressive disorder, anorexia nervosa and obsessive disorders, and by historical convention, pervasive developmental disorders such as autism.

In clinical practice, these terms are not universally adopted. In particular, many clinicians think it is inappropriate to label preschool children as having mental disorders, and prefer to describe young children, in their family and social context, by compiling a list of problems and strengths.[5] Typical mental health problems in those aged 0–5 can be conveniently grouped into two main categories, although many individual children will have problems of both sorts.

Behaviour problems

Transient behaviour problems are almost universal in toddlers and preschoolers, but may sometimes become more established, troublesome and extreme in comparison with other children of the same developmental level.

Typical behaviour problems include:

- marked disobedience, aggression, and temper tantrums;
- excessive restlessness, inattentiveness, and impulsiveness;
- sleeping and feeding problems.

119

Emotional problems

Children with emotional problems may seem exceptionally withdrawn, tearful, unhappy or anxious in comparison with their peers of a similar age. They might appear preoccupied by worries or fears, or develop phobias.

Children with multiple problems in either or both categories are particularly important to identify as they are at increased risk of persistent mental health problems. Another group worth identifying by school entry are the 2–3% of children who are exceptionally restless, inattentive, and impulsive. Most preschoolers are restless, inattentive and impulsive to some degree, but for a small percentage of those children at the extreme end of the spectrum, their symptoms are sufficiently severe to regard them as having hyperkinetic disorder or attention deficit hyperactivity disorder (ADHD). These diagnoses have been the subject of much controversy. Until recently different diagnostic criteria were in use in America and Britain, and some clinicians were more willing to make the diagnosis than others. However appropriate diagnosis in severely affected children is important, as early identification can access effective specialist treatment, without which they are likely to end up with associated educational and behavioural problems.

Because young children are so particularly dependent on their families for care and stimulation, it is essential to think of their problems in a family context. Young children's mental health problems can often arise out of difficulties within the family. Where they do not, the ability of the family to manage the problems is crucial in determining their overall impact. A young child's problems often affect everybody in the family, directly or indirectly, and the capacity of the family to function effectively will also be affected by their local community and the wider cultural and political context. This interdependency is illustrated in Figure 7.1.

The other exceptional characteristic of the 0–5 age group is the extraordinarily rapid pace of their development, making it especially

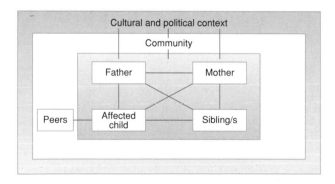

Fig 7.1   The child's family and wider context

important to take developmental issues into consideration. Children with developmental delays and deviations are particularly prone to mental health problems. These can arise where a child has one isolated developmental delay, for example in speech and language, or else where children have impairments in multiple aspects of their development such as autism. It is important both to consider unrecognised developmental delay as a potential cause of emotional and behaviour problems in 0–5s, and also to monitor children with known developmental delays and deviations closely for associated mental health problems.

Prevalence and patterns in mental health problems in children aged 0–5

Prevalence

One survey of the prevalence of mental health problems in young children living in an Outer London Borough found that 7% of 3 year olds had moderate or severe behaviour problems, with a further 15% having mild problems. The term "behaviour problems" included, for example, frequent sleep disturbance, excessive fears or worries, soiling, and excessive overactivity.[6] This study is particularly informative because it provides longitudinal data, reinterviewing parents of children who had had behaviour problems at age 3, again at age 4, and age 8. A control group who had not had behaviour problems at age 3 was interviewed at the same ages.

Table 7.1 shows some changes in prevalence in various problems over time.

These percentages in Table 7.1 indicate that, at a population level, "being difficult to control" shows a striking persistence over time. Levels of fears, soiling, comfort habits and night waking all decline sharply between the

Table 7.1   Percentage of children with specific problems at different ages

Specific problems	3 years	4 years	8 years
Fears	10	12	2
Overactive, restless	17	13	11
Worries	4	10	21
Difficult to control	11	10	11
Soiling (> 1/week)	16	3	4
Many comfort habits	17	14	1
Waking at night (> 3/week)	14	12	3
Poor appetite	19	20	13

$n = 705$; of these, 101 problem children, 101 controls and 10 language group children were intensively investigated with further interviews and testing.
(Source: Richman N, Stevenson J, Graham PJ. *Preschool to School: a behavioural study.* London: Academic Press, 1982)

121

ages of 3 and 8. Levels of overactive restlessness and poor appetite decline to some extent. Worries become much more prominent as the children get older, presumably reflecting greater cognitive sophistication.

There were some other interesting findings in this study. At age 3, there were slightly more problems in boys, who were more hyperactive, while girls were more fearful. Mental health problems were more common in the presence of specific language delay, marital discord, low warmth, high criticism, maternal depression, large family size, and high rise housing.

When the children were revisited at 8 years old, it was found that of the 3 year olds with problems, 73% of boys still had problems, as did 48% of girls. Overactivity and low intelligence predicted persistence of problems in boys but not in girls. Overactivity predicted conduct disorder, and fearfulness predicted emotional disorder.

Data from the same study were analysed to determine the level of behaviour problems in 3 year old children of West Indian born parents. No difference was found between levels of behaviour problems in this group and in the indigenous sample.[7]

Long-term outcome of mental health problems in children aged 0–5

There is now good evidence that problems in the early years of childhood may presage problems in adolescence and adult life. A New Zealand longitudinal study of mental health outcomes showed that restless impulsive 3 year olds had higher rates of serious persistent antisocial behaviour at age 21, and unduly shy, inhibited 3 year olds had higher rates of depression at the same age. Three year old boys in either group had an increased risk of alcohol related problems at age 21, and both groups of 3 year olds had an increased risk of suicide during adolescence.[2] Another review concluded that children identified as hard to manage at ages 3 or 4 have a high probability (probably somewhere around 50:50) of continuing to show difficulties throughout the elementary school years and into adolescence.[8]

This review identified the following factors as predictive of behaviour problems which persist from the early years:

• the presence of multiple behaviour difficulties (spread);
• problems evident in different contexts (pervasiveness);
• a distressed and/or dysfunctional family context.

Physical punishment at home has also been linked with ongoing and increased behaviour problems, impaired learning, delinquency, and aggression.[9] This is particularly worrying given the general statistic that 90% of UK children have been hit in some form.[10]

The potentially adverse long–term consequences of emotional and behavioural problems in early childhood mean that these should merit identification and treatment in the preschool years.[11] However, young children and families deserve help and treatment not only to prevent problems arising later on, but also to alleviate their current distress.

Risk and protective factors for young children's mental health problems

Children's mental health problems are not the product of simple chains of causality. Apparently similar problems may have arisen for very different reasons in different children. For example, in children whose main problem is aggressive behaviour, this may have a number of different causes. For some, their aggression may be linked to their individual characteristics. In children with delayed language development, they may hit out because their limited powers of communication leave them frustrated. In other children, family issues may be more important. Domestic violence within the family may be echoed by aggression in the children. Yet for others, social issues may have a significant impact. In families where unemployment, poor housing and financial difficulties combine to preoccupy the adults, there may be little time and energy available for appropriate parenting. For many children with mental health problems, individual, family and social risk factors such as these will interact. In the same way that there is little specificity linking children's mental health problems with single causative factors, in general, there is also a lack of specificity between particular risk factors and particular mental health problems in children.

Single risk factors are less powerfully correlated with mental disorder in children than multiple risk factors. Having a single risk factor very slightly increases the risk of having a disorder, and having two to three risk factors increases the risk a little more, but having four or more risk factors make it much more likely that a child will develop a mental disorder. One study identified five variables which cumulatively prove to be significantly associated with psychiatric disorder in children: severe marital discord; low social status; overcrowding or large family size, paternal criminality; and maternal psychiatric disorder. By contrast, only 6% with two or three factors, and those with a single factor, had a barely increased risk of psychiatric disorder.[12]

In conceptualising causation in individual cases, it is useful to think of a balance between risk factors and protective factors. Protective factors can reduce the adverse impact of risk factors. For example, a single mother with a low income may find the support of her extended family helps her cope with her new baby, and protects her from the normal ups and downs of new motherhood becoming chronically problematical.

Table 7.2 categorises some risk and protective factors. It is not exhaustive.

123

Table 7.2   Child, family and social risk factors for mental health problems in children

Social	Family	Child
	Risk factors	
Socio–economic disadvantage	Poor parenting skills	Genetic influences
Homelessness	Abuse	Difficult temperament
Isolation	Marital discord	Chronic physical or
	Family breakdown through divorce or death	neurological illness
	Parental mental illness	Low IQ
	Large families	Specific developmental delays
		Communication difficulties
	Protective factors	
Family friendly government policies	Affection	Easy temperament
Social support	Supervision	High self–esteem
Adequate standard of living	Promotion of self–esteem	
Access to good quality child care	Authoritative discipline	

(Adapted from: Health Advisory Service. *Child and Adolescent Mental Health Services: together we stand.* London: HMSO, 1995. © Crown Copyright material is reproduced with the permission of the Controller of Her Majesty's Stationery Office)

It is important to emphasise again the interactive nature of these risk and protective factors.

Social risk and protective factors

Socio–economic disadvantage

Children in social classes IV and V have an increased risk of mortality, compared to children in social classes I and II.[13] They also have increased levels of morbidity.[14] Mental disorders in children do not show this marked class differential, and overall these disorders are not more common in low income groups.[15] Conduct disorder (an ICD10/DSMIVR diagnosis involving persistent antisocial, aggressive or defiant behaviour) is an exception, as it is more common in social classes IV and V, and in younger children is associated with low family income. But in general, although there are many good reasons for attempting to eradicate poverty, it may not be realistic to expect that a reduction in poverty levels would bring with it a substantial reduction in emotional and behavioural problems and subsequent psychiatric disorder.

Poverty is often only one of many challenges facing disadvantaged families, who may also have to cope with poor housing or homelessness, unsafe environments, inadequate local amenities and poor nutrition.[16] How well a family manages to function in the face of chronically debilitating problems like these will influence the degree to which socio–economic adversity affects their children's mental health. These chronic adversities are characteristically (but not exclusively) associated with inner city life. In inner cities, high concentrations of ethnic minority families may be further disadvantaged by lack of access to services and the insidious effects of racism.[17] Refugees, with the additional psychological stress of an enforced move to an unfamiliar society, and an uncertain future, are also likely to live in conditions of multiple adversity, with a consequent impact on their children's mental health.[18]

Housing and homelessness

There is good evidence that inadequate housing has an adverse effect on children's mental health. Overcrowding has been identified as a variable which, alongside other risk factors, is associated with increased rates of psychiatric disorder in children.[12] One study[19] found that mothers in high–rise accommodation had increased levels of maternal depression, which is linked to behaviour problems and poor cognitive performance in children. Homeless families have also been identified as a group with particular mental health needs which are often unmet. A longitudinal study of homeless families found high levels of mental health problems in homeless children and their mothers, which persisted in a substantial minority after rehousing.[20]

Social isolation and social support

The birth of a baby, especially a first child, involves a considerable number of social and psychological adjustments on the part of both parents.[21, 22] This transition can be facilitated by the support of kin and community networks, which can have a protective effect.

Developing a social support structure, often among parents themselves, or using volunteers, is a prominent feature of many initiatives intended to improve parenting skills and children's health. However it is important to remember that parents are active participants in the creation of their own social environments, and those parents most likely to abuse or neglect their children may be least likely to develop and utilise community support networks.[23] These parents will need long–term multidisciplinary pro-fessional support to develop and maintain their parenting skills. But short–term interventions at key times with vulnerable groups can also be worthwhile. A follow-up study of mothers at high risk for low birthweight, who had had a programme of social support in pregnancy, found at follow-up when the children were aged 7 that there were fewer behaviour problems among the children and less anxiety among the mothers in the intervention group.[24]

Family risk and protective factors

Research evidence suggests that, in general, it is not the structure of a family which will determine whether children develop mental health problems, but how that family functions. There are some associations linking large family size and certain family structures with increased mental health problems, but these are best understood as indicative of associated risk factors, such as lack of individual parental attention.

Children from large families are twice as likely to develop conduct disorder and become delinquent than children from smaller families.[25] Such children are also more likely to have delayed language development, lower verbal intelligence and lower reading attainment, and experience less parental supervision and more sibling aggression, all of which may contribute to their behaviour problems.[26]

Children living in single parent families have increased rates of emotional, behavioural and educational difficulties,[27] but this increased risk is not sustained when poverty is taken into account.[28] Children raised in lesbian families are not at increased risk of mental health problems.[29]

Quality of parenting

It is often the quality of parenting available in a family, as they tackle the normal or exceptional problems of their child's development, which differentiates between a difficult child who develops mental health problems and a difficult child who achieves his or her potential. A family's capacity to parent effectively will be intimately connected to the levels of support and stress they experience. How parents raise their children is influenced not only by how they were raised themselves and who they become, but also by the everyday circumstances of their lives, and the resources to which they have access.[30] Statutory and voluntary services can play an important role in helping parents provide a nurturing environment for their children.

Parenting begins before birth and the developing fetus can be affected by smoking, drugs (including alcohol), and excessive maternal stress or anxiety. Smoking in pregnancy increases the risk of low birthweight, with its attendant problems. If the developing fetus is regularly exposed to heroin, cocaine or large amounts of alcohol, a variety of adverse effects have been reported, including short- and long–term difficulties with modulating arousal, activity level, and attention.[31] These deficits can make parenting difficult, and where the parent is still involved in substance abuse, they may already have reduced resources for the task of parenting. Pregnancy may, however, act as a trigger for behavioural change, inspired by concern for the developing fetus. Advice, sensitively given, may help pregnant mothers reduce their alcohol intake, stop smoking, and using other drugs. Excessive maternal stress and anxiety have also been shown to be linked with prematurity and low birthweight.[32] Some studies,[33, 34] but not others,[35] suggest that these adverse effects can be reduced by preventive interventions in pregnancy.

From birth onwards, parents develop a repertoire of practical parenting skills, derived from their own experience of being parented, advice from kin and community networks, and social and cultural norms.

Research into parenting has established many models. One model developed by Maccoby and Martin identified four styles with different outcomes for the future mental health and functioning of children along two different dimensions, level of demand/control versus level of acceptance/rejection.[36]

Authoritarian parenting

Children growing up in authoritarian families, with high levels of demand and control but relatively low levels of warmth or acceptance, tend to be less socially skilled, do not internalise standards of good behaviour and have lower self–esteem. Some of these children may appear subdued; others may show high aggressiveness or other indications of being out of control.[37]

Permissive parenting

Children growing up with indulgent or permissive parents, who are warm but provide low levels of demand and control, also show some negative outcomes, and by adolescence tend to be more aggressive, immature, irresponsible, and lacking in independence.[38]

Neglecting parenting

Neglecting parents provide neither warmth and acceptance nor adequate demand and control. Their children tend to show disturbances in their relationships with peers and with adults for many years. At adolescence, for example, youngsters from neglecting families are more impulsive and antisocial, less competent with their peers, and much less achievement oriented in school.[39]

Authoritative parenting

These parents provide high levels of both control and warmth, setting clear limits but also responding to the child's individual needs. Their children typically show higher self–esteem, and are more independent, are more likely to comply with parental requests, and may show more altruistic behaviour as well. They are self–confident and achieve greater educational success.[39]

The limitation of this type of classificatory approach to parenting is that it can appear to play down the impact of contextual and child factors. It is important to stress that parent–child relationships are not simply the result of the adult's parenting style. Children with difficult temperaments will tend to elicit authoritarian parenting, while children with easier tempera- ments will be easier to parent in an authoritative way.[40] In some circumstances, parenting is almost inevitably disrupted. Children are at an increased risk of mental health problems where there is parental dis- harmony or divorce or separation. Each family situation is different and no universal recommendation can be made about whether parents in conflict should stay together or split up. The relative merits of each course of action, and the wishes of all family members, including the children, should be taken into account. For families facing divorce or separation, or coping with the death of a parent, the young children will benefit from minimal disruptions to their usual routine, a simple explanation of what is happening, and reassurance that it is not their fault. There is plenty of evidence that parents who are warm and affectionate, in the context of clear, firm limit–setting, will have a positive impact on their children's mental health. This is the basis for a wide variety of parent education initiatives.

Physical punishment

Physical punishment or smacking a child is often perceived as an effective child care practice in disciplining a child. However, with increasing research attention on this subject, evidence is accumulating to suggest otherwise. Children often learn most effectively by example, and smacking provides the example that problems should be solved by resorting to physical aggression. Smacking is therefore a lesson in bad behaviour rather than good behaviour and can increase the likelihood of violent and aggressive behaviour in the long term.[41] The first meta–analysis of physical punish- ment, covering 88 studies, is soon to be published. The results show, with unusual consistency, that although corporal punishment does secure children's immediate compliance, it also increases the likelihood of negative outcomes.[42] Following the recent hearing in the European Court of Human Rights, the UK government is now clarifying British law concerning the physical punishment of children by parents and their delegates.[43]

Child abuse

Emotional abuse is defined as "actual or likely severe adverse effects on the emotional and behavioural development of a child caused by persistent or severe emotional ill–treatment or rejection".[44] Young children who are being or have been emotionally abused may have a whole range of mental health problems, including defiance and aggression, apparent depression, lack of interest in learning, and disturbed relationships with adults. Children who have been physically, sexually or emotionally abused are sometimes found to show "frozen watchfulness" as though anticipating further abuse. Sexually abused young children may become involved in sexually explicit play with their friends or be sexually provocative with adults.[45] Many, but not all abused children will have longer-term mental health problems. If the childhood abuse has not resulted in death or disability, in the long term it is the psychological components of the early abuse which contributes most to adverse outcomes.[46] A proportion (around 30%) of adults abused as children will go on to abuse their own children,[47] and their risk of depression in adulthood is much increased.

The focus of child protection must not only be on identification of existing abuse, but also on family support to reduce the likelihood of abuse occurring in the first place.

Parental mental disorder (including postnatal depression)

Parental mental disorder may also be associated with increased rates of mental disorder in children. This is often assumed to be because the mental disorder disrupts effective parenting, but may also be because of a shared genetic vulnerability between parent and child, or because the child is exposed to many other environmental adversities such as poverty, poor housing and isolation, which are often features of life for those with chronic mental illness. The types of disorder which children develop do not correspond exactly to those experienced by their parents, though there is a tendency for young children of depressed mothers to show apparent symptoms of depression, and an association between personality disorder in a parent and conduct disorder in children.[48] Parents with mental illnesses may be consistently or periodically affected, and their parenting can be severely, or only mildly affected. Where they are unable to parent effectively, the effect on their children can be buffered by the presence of another adult, or the other parent, who can take on the main caregiving role as necessary, ideally with minimum disruption to the children's normal routines.

For children aged 0–5 years, one important category of parental mental illness which has been the subject of much research is postnatal depression. This affects approximately 10% of mothers. Many mothers with postnatal depression find it difficult to provide sensitive and responsive care for their infants, and observational studies have shown both behavioural and physiological changes in the infants of these mothers.[33]

As postnatal depression is common, and both a simple screening instrument and effective treatments are available,[49] a universal screening and early intervention programme delivered by health visitors and general practitioners is feasible, effective, and desirable.[50] Recent studies have suggested that fathers may also experience some degree of depression after the birth of a child.[51] Postnatal depression is a condition for which a secondary preventive model is unlikely to be optimum.

Non–parental care: day care, fostering, and adoption

Child care

For many parents, finding child care while they work is a necessity. This may be provided in various ways within and outside the home, such as by members of the extended family, childminders, nurseries, nannies, and au pairs. There is no evidence that non–parental care of adequate quality is harmful to the mental health of children. In fact quality day care can provide cognitive advantages for children from disadvantaged homes.[52] Several studies have found that for children under 1 year of age in non–maternal care for more than 5 hours there is a small increased risk of insecure attachment, though the interpretation and implications of this finding have been the subject of much debate.[53]

Good quality day care is characterised by high staff–child ratios, individualised rather than institutionalised care, effective key worker systems, good staff–parent communication, child oriented verbal inter-action, and the provision of varied activities within a structured day. Similar features can be used to evaluate the quality of other non–parental care arrangements such as childminders or nannies.

Fostering and adoption

In the design and delivery of community child health services, it is often assumed that parents are the best monitors of child health and are able to seek appropriate advice. Children in public care may lack a powerful advocate to negotiate the continuance of any health input arranged in their "home" area. There can be delay in meeting their educational needs with consequent behavioural, emotional and learning consequences (Miles M, personal communication, 1998).

For adults who were fostered long term, adopted, or brought up in an institution (children in public care), the personal and social outcomes are most favourable among those who were adopted and least favourable among those brought up in institutions, with those in long–term fostering in an intermediate position.[54] All these groups of children are at increased risk of mental health problems. The widespread belief that early adoption is much more likely to be successful, because the child will benefit from stable early relationships with the adoptive parents remains broadly true, but research shows that later adoptions can also work well.[55] There is a trend to place children where possible with extended family, and also for open adoptions, with contact between the adoptive and biological families. The psychological impact of open adoption has yet to be fully researched. The debate about cross-cultural adoption continues, though it is widely agreed that children should not be allowed to remain in institutional or short-term foster care if a racially matched adoption can not be achieved but good adoptive care is otherwise available.[56] Fostering and adoption are more likely to work for the mutual benefit of carers and children where care is taken in establishing the initial placements, and the families have specialised support and help available when they need it.

Individual risk factors

Genetic factors

The old debate over whether particular mental health problems arise because of nature (genetics) or nurture (environment) has been replaced by a much more sophisticated appreciation that genes and environment act in a way which is mutually interlinked. A child's genetic inheritance may contribute a vulnerability which, in combination with environmental adversity, can result in mental health problems.

The relative contributions of genetics and environment vary between different conditions. For example, conduct disorder is largely the product of environment, while autism is predominantly determined genetically. Therapeutic and environmental interventions remain important for both genetically and environmentally determined disorders. Microchip based gene probes are currently in development which may enable the early identification of risk factors for later psychological development, such as the genetic predisposition for inattention and restlessness. If these gene probes become commercially available, it is important that children identified as high risk should be the recipients of environmental and therapeutic assistance rather than discrimination (Hill P, personal communication, 1988).

Disability

Children with a variety of disabilities are known to be at increased risk of mental health problems. Approximately one-third of children with mild

Table 7.3 Increased risk of psychiatric disorders in children with physical disabilities: results from an epidemiological study of 10–11 year olds

	% with psychiatric disorder
No physical disorder	7
Physical disorder not affecting the brain	12
Idiopathic epilepsy	29
Cerebral palsy and allied disorders: IQ > 70	44

(Source: Goodman R, Scott S. *Child Psychiatry*. Oxford: Blackwell Science, 1997. Reproduced with permission from the publishers)

learning disabilities have psychiatric diagnoses, as do roughly half of all children with severe learning disabilities. This compares with some 10–15% of other children judged by the same criteria. The children with mild learning disabilities have similar types of psychiatric disorders as other children, but children with severe retardation are more likely to have autistic type syndromes, hyperactivity, self–injurious behaviour, and sleep problems.

Children with physical disabilities are also at increased risk of psychiatric disorders, particularly where their disability involves brain damage. Table 7.3 shows relevant results from an epidemiological study of 10 and 11 year olds.

Other disabilities in children have also been shown to be associated with increased rates of psychiatric disturbance, including severe hearing loss[57] and marked language delay or impairment.[58]

The increased rates of mental health problems in children with disabilities is in some cases related to brain damage, and in others linked to the psychosocial disadvantages experienced by some disabled children. Many children will have both a biological and psychosocial vulnerability to mental health problems. For families, it is often the behavioural problems like chronically disturbed sleep or aggressive outbursts which are the hardest aspects of their child's problems to deal with.

One approach to primary prevention of emotional and behavioural problems linked to childhood disability involves strategies to reduce the numbers of children born with, or developing disabilities. On the one hand, antenatal screening and selective termination has resulted in some babies with disabilities not being born. On the other hand, developments in special care for premature babies have led to the survival of babies with physical handicaps and learning disabilities who would previously have died.

The families of these babies and also those whose children's disabilities become apparent at a later stage, need a comprehensive range of support which may involve health, education, social and voluntary services. Improving the early detection of emotional and behavioural problems in disabled children and the effective management of these problems involves developing greater awareness and skills among professionals and others involved with these families.

Attachment

Attachment theory, as proposed by Bowlby[59-61] and modified since, has stimulated an extensive body of research, much of which has implications for young children's mental health. Bowlby's clear exposition of the importance of facilitating young children's developing attachments to their main caregivers has underpinned many important developments in child care practice for those aged 0–5. Young children are no longer admitted to hospitals without their parents, nurseries and day care facilities (in principle at least) use keyworkers with whom children are encouraged to develop special relationships, and adoptions are, where possible, completed while children are young.

Children's attachments can be classified in four ways: secure, insecure avoidant, insecure ambivalent, and disorganised. Insecure attachments are associated with a number of disadvantages in psychosocial development.

Children classified as having disorganised attachments often come from families which face marked socio–economic adversities, may have parents with major problems like abuse[62] or severe depression,[63] or themselves be the victims of abuse.[64] These children are at greatly increased risk of having preschool behaviour problems,[65] though it is likely that their disorganised attachment status is only one element in an array of risk factors to which they have been exposed. Insecure and disorganised attachments are only risk factors for future adverse outcomes, and not mental disorders in their own right. But some children will have such marked abnormalities in their relationships with their caregivers and develop such aberrant behaviour patterns that they can be regarded as having attachment disorders.[66, 67]

Those children who have typically spent their early years in poor quality institutional care, will tend to have long-term problems with social functioning, even when adopted into more favourable circumstances,[68] though adoption is likely to be the best available alternative for them.

The discussion above has demonstrated that there are numerous risk factors for mental health problems in those aged 0–5, and children who are growing up with several of these risk factors are much more likely to develop mental health problems than children exposed to single risk factors. Some children will be protected from developing problems by virtue of their individual characteristics. These include qualities which are predominantly genetically determined, such as easy temperament or high IQ. Other attributes such as secure attachments, positive self–image, effective interpersonal skills, cognitive skills and the development of special talents, can be nurtured through good parenting. The need for service provision will vary from family to family, but for some, it is likely that preventive interventions need to be provided long term, in what has been described as a "nutritional" manner, rather than on a one off "inoculation" basis.[69] This underlines the importance of developing, at national and local levels, integrated policies and intervention strategies for families with children of all ages.

Interventions to reduce mental health problems

At a local level many services and sectors contribute to promoting young children's mental health. The four main services and sectors involved are primary and secondary (specialised) health care, education services, social services, and the voluntary sector, but children's mental health will also be influenced by the adequacy of other local services, including council housing policy, provision for homeless families, parks, libraries, leisure services, etc. Specialist child and adolescent mental health services (CAMHS) may be more or less involved with this age group, depending on local patterns of service. The box on the next page shows the structural framework within which CAMHS are planned, and describes typical contributions of specialist child mental health services to mental health promotion and early intervention with children aged 0–5.[3]

Although the importance of interagency collaboration in promoting young children's mental health has been reiterated for years, unfortunately it is difficult to organise a review of current interventions except by dividing up those interventions along agency lines. There is, in general, little interagency work to blur the boundaries. For that reason, selected samples of contributions from health care, social services, education and the voluntary sector will be considered in turn. The provision of parenting education will then be reviewed.

Effective interventions within health care

Routine antenatal care and child health surveillance provide an ideal opportunity for the promotion of young children's mental health. Health visitors, with their particular remit to identify health care needs in those aged 0–5, are central to this screening process, but their role is currently the subject of debate, with job losses in some health authorities.[70] With the proposed targeting of health visitor input to the most needy children and families, and not all children and families, it is important that families understand their responsibility in initiating contact when they have concerns. Many families await health visitor contact before sharing concern. The development of primary care groups should provide better opportunities for both effective identification and intervention.

Tier 1: Primary or direct contact services

Workers in this tier include GPs, health visitors, voluntary sector workers, social workers, nursery workers, etc. These workers influence children's mental health as an aspect of, rather than the primary purpose of, their work. They may be involved in aspects of mental health promotion, explicitly or otherwise, and are well placed to identify and help many children with mental health problems, or their families, without referring to specialist services. They can be supported in doing this more effectively through training and supervision.

Tier 2: Interventions offered by individual specialist child and adolescent mental health professionals

In this tier, individual professionals with specialist mental health training work may work directly with young children and their families, or supervise and train those in Tier 1. These individuals may have a variety of professional qualifications in, for example, psychology, psychiatry, social work, and psychotherapy. A community psychiatric nurse or a psychotherapist offering supervision to health visitors, a psychiatrist providing regular consultation in a special needs nursery, or a clinical psychologist running a clinic for sleep and behaviour problems are examples of ways in which Tier 2 professionals might be involved in promoting mental health in the 0–5s. The appointment of specialist child mental health workers with a specific remit to provide consultations and outreach work in Tier 1 has been introduced in some areas. Paediatricians working in child development clinics also provide a specialist service at this level for young children, especially those with developmental delay and associated behavioural problems.

Tier 3. Interventions offered by teams of staff from specialist child and adolescent mental health services

Professionals in this tier may have similar backgrounds to those in Tier 2, but work in co-ordinated teams with client families, rather than individually. They offer integrated multidisciplinary assessment and management. Unless particular teams have a special interest relating to younger children and their families, much work at Tier 3 may be focused on school age children and adolescents.

Tier 4: very specialised interventions and care

Work in this tier relates to highly specific and complex problems, including for example, services for children with eating disorders, autism or other pervasive developmental disorders.

The priority given to the prevention of children's mental health problems by GPs and health visitors is variable. Where some priority is given innovative projects can be developed.

A general practice in Dorset used GP fundholding growth money to finance a "Child and Family Counsellor" who works in an exceptionally flexible way. The postholder had training in family therapy and experience of working with seriously disturbed children. Referrals are accepted from primary health care colleagues, teachers, social workers, and also children and families themselves. Children, alone or with their families, are seen at school, in the surgery or at home. Interventions may also address issues between child and school, family and school, or between agencies. Feedback from parents and referrers has been very positive.[71]

Aside from innovative initiatives of this sort, there are three main ways in which primary care professionals, or other interested professionals and voluntary workers can develop their interests in this field:

- by developing supervision and consultation arrangements with local psychologists, psychiatrists or psychotherapists;
- by extending their expertise through individual training;
- by participating in locality–wide initiatives – these types of programmes mainly involve health visitors, and all or many health visitors in an area are trained to deliver a specific intervention.

Four approaches are described below:

Strategies for identifying and treating postnatal depression

Postnatal depression, if it persists, is associated with a number of adverse effects in the infant. Reducing the levels of postnatal depression in a community is likely to have a positive effect on the children of those mothers whose depression is identified and treated. A validated screening instrument is available: the Edinburgh Postnatal Depression Scale or EPDS.[49] Treatment for postnatal depression may involve antidepressants, but there is also good evidence for the efficacy of non–directive counselling in some cases. A randomised controlled trial demonstrated that after eight health visitor "listening visits", 69% of the depressed women who were counselled recovered from their depression, compared to 38% of those in the control group.[72] Many areas have now introduced a protocol training health visitors in the use of the EPDS, and in non–directive counselling, with clear guidelines for involving GPs and psychiatric services where mothers do not benefit from a counselling intervention.

The Child Development Programme

This programme, developed at Bristol University, involves specially trained health visitors in regular semi-structured home visits which focus specifically on empowering parents, and use information sheets with illustrative cartoons to promote effective parenting and aspects of child development.

The programme is usually targeted towards first time parents during the first year of their child's life, or parents who are having difficulties with their older preschool children. Although the Child Development Programme has not been subject to rigorous evaluation against a control group, families receiving the intervention have been shown to have high levels of immunisation uptake, less hospitalisation of infants, low levels of child abuse, and an improved home environment. The Child Development Programme is in use in at least 25 Trusts across Britain.[73]

The Parent Adviser Service

This service has been developed in a highly deprived area of South London. It involves health visitors and community medical officers, given a brief training in parent counselling skills, parenting issues and behavioural management, visiting families with young children who are asking for help in managing aspects of their children's behaviour. The health visitors work with the parents, using a counselling approach to explore ways of tackling the presenting problems and others that arise in discussion.

An evaluation of the service found at least short–term improvements in the children's problems, and raised self–esteem, less depression and less stress for the mothers. There was also an improvement in the children's home environment. However, longer-term effectiveness remains to be assessed.[74]

A more unusual approach which may be a blueprint for primary care services of the future is illustrated in the following example, where health services are provided in partnership with services from other agencies and the voluntary sector.

Bromley by Bow Centre

This centre, in a highly deprived area of East London, is funded from the Single Regeneration Budget, local and national businesses, National Lottery money, and donations from charities. It organises activities in seven main areas: art, Bengali outreach, community care, employment, health, park, and youth. It has recently designed and built its own health centre, where three GPs, other health professionals, artists and community project workers will offer an integrated range of clinical and other services to local people.[75]

Effective interventions within social services

While primary care professionals have particular routine opportunities to identify children with mental health problems, or families likely to develop such problems, social services, in conjunction with health, education and voluntary agencies, are important service providers for such families. Social services have a dual role, with responsibilities for child protection and also for family support, and in both these capacities can have a positive effect on young children's mental health. The Children Act (1989) encouraged a reorientation of social services away from an exclusive concentration on detection of cases of suspected abuse and neglect, towards a balance between protection and preventive provision for vulnerable families. Local authorities were charged with a duty to "safeguard and promote the welfare of children within their area who are in need by providing a range and level of services appropriate to those children's needs". "In need" was defined in terms of children disabled physically, emotionally or mentally, or whose physical, emotional or mental development was impaired or likely to be impaired. How far the shift from child protection towards preventive provision for vulnerable families has occurred varies very much around the country.[76]

Typical social service provision of support to vulnerable families includes family centres and drop–ins. One study concluded that open access family centres appear to be effective in promoting family well-being,[77] but these types of centre may not be used by those families most in need. The importance of developing non-stigmatising, accessible community-based family support facilities cannot be overestimated. The opportunities for joint funding and planning with education and the voluntary sector are obvious.

Sandal Agbrigg Pre–five Centre, Wakefield, Yorkshire

The funding of this combined nursery and family support centre is equally shared between the Education and Social Services Departments in Wakefield. It has a mixed catchment area, and provides part–time nursery education for 3–5 year olds, with on–site developmental checks and speech therapy. There is also a programme of family support for families where a child has special needs or there are parenting difficulties, including child protection issues. Parents are also offered a variety of adult education classes, and some respite care of younger children. There has been no formal evaluation of the effectiveness of the preventive work at this centre, but there is a local consensus that fewer families have been placed on the child protection register as a result of the help with parenting that they have received, and children are well prepared to begin their school education. Evaluation of this scheme should be conducted and the monitoring of the number of children on the Child Protection Register could be easily verifiable as an outcome. Unfortunately, this integrated service has proven expensive and more work needs to be done on running integrated services in a way which does not send costs spiralling.[78]

Effective interventions within education services

Preschool education provides an opportunity for promoting young children's mental health, and identifying children with emotional and behavioural problems so that they and their families can find help. Good quality preschool provision promotes cognitive, physical, social and emotional development in tandem. Evidence from American preschool programmes for disadvantaged children points to long–term benefits in a variety of domains. The following example has been the most extensively evaluated.

High Scope

This preschool curriculum was developed in the 1960s in Ypsilanti, Michigan, as one of many Head Start initiatives funded by the US government in an attempt to improve educational achievements for children in low income families. High Scope encourages active learning, with children planning activities, carrying them out, and then reviewing their outcomes. The evaluated High Scope programme involved 2.5 hour sessions for 5 days of the week, where children worked with trained adults, in groups of six children per adult. The programme also included weekly 1.5 hour home visits where the children's progress was discussed with parents. Longitudinal studies to age 27 compared a group of 123 disadvantaged children who had had 2 years of the High Scope programme with a similar group who did not attend preschool, and found a number of statistically significant differences. The studies found that more of the High Scope group had completed their high school education, that they had had fewer arrests, fewer teenage pregnancies, higher employment rates, better salaries, more further education, less use of social services, and higher levels of home ownership. The cost of the High Scope programme was a little over $12,000 per child, and it has been estimated that more than $88,000 was saved per participant in terms of less need for special education, savings on welfare and criminal justice costs, savings on settlements for victims of crimes, and more taxes paid on higher incomes.[79]

When the outcomes of several different initiatives under the Head Start programme were pooled, it was found that though initial increases in IQ had faded after 3 or 4 years, children who had attended high quality preschool provision were less likely to need special education or be held back a grade, and were more likely to be in employment.[80]

High Scope has been the most extensively evaluated preschool curriculum. Debate continues over whether it offers unique benefits, or whether it shares many elements in common with other high quality preschool programmes.[81] These common elements include staffing stability, high staff/child ratio, children from a range of socio–economic backgrounds, close links with parents, child-centred active learning, careful records of children's progress, and adequate time for staff training, supervision, and reflection. High Scope is being introduced and evaluated in a number of British nursery schools.

Although preschool education programmes have generally been evaluated in terms of cognitive and social outcomes, it is likely that individuals successful in these areas also have good self–esteem, and fewer emotional and behavioural problems. In fact strategies likely to promote cognitive and social development will often be beneficial in terms of mental health. For example, with young babies an emphasis on sensitive responsiveness to the infant's communicative cues is likely to promote both language development and secure attachment between the child and his or her parent. In toddlers and preschoolers, promoting a judicious combination of warm encouragement, exploration and limit setting as part of any educational initiative is also likely to benefit both cognitive development and mental health. Guiding preschool children through tasks which are sufficiently, but not excessively taxing, is likely to encourage both problem solving skills and a sense of competence and self–esteem. In addition, good quality day care, nursery provision or childminding, where well trained carers work in partnership with parents, can often be a source of advice and support for parents, who may benefit from observing alternative child rearing practices.

The current government has placed education at the top of their list of priorities, and explains many of their new initiatives for those aged 0–5 in terms of preparation for learning at school. The move towards nursery care and education for 3 year olds and the development of more extensive, affordable, quality child care provision are in fact likely to bring both educational and mental health benefits, particularly to children facing multiple adversities. The benefits to children from higher socio–economic groups will depend on the quality of preschool provision or child care relative to the quality of the experience available to them at home.

Monitoring and improving the quality of education and child care for young children is essential. The education service has a responsibility for monitoring the quality of early education and day care, and the way in which this should be achieved is currently under review. This is particularly important given the planned expansion in child care for those aged 0–5. Alongside improving regulation and standard setting, the government also plans to encourage more extensive training for nursery workers, day care workers and childminders, although decisions on minimum standards have not yet been made.

To maximise the beneficial effects of preschool education on children facing multiple adversities, evidence suggests that it is crucial that good practice is not simply confined to the nursery premises, but that efforts are made to involve parents at every stage. How far parents can develop their parenting skills and raise their expectations for their children, will alter their children's home environment with effects lasting years after the preschool period.

Effective interventions in the voluntary sector

The voluntary sector, and user groups of patients, carers or disabled people have been influential in innovative thinking on health care, access to appropriate health care, and rethinking service provision to take account of the perspectives of users. The voluntary sector provides many services for those aged under five and their families, including playgroups and nurseries. Many of these services are small scale responses to local needs, and may develop out of the work of existing organisations such as churches or community groups. These small groups may often find themselves able to deliver services which are particularly responsive to local needs, and seen as non–stigmatising by families. The downside of this freedom is greater uncertainty about continued funding. In addition, volunteers providing services to families may have less access to training and expertise, and they are not necessarily subject to the same levels of quality control as professional workers. However not all voluntary sector initiatives are small scale. There are some larger voluntary sector family support services with well established programmes, where trained volunteers deliver effective interventions to families with young children. Some of these programmes, and their evaluations are reviewed below.

Homestart

Homestart is a befriending service which was started in Leicester in 1973. By 1992 it was operating in 130 urban and rural areas, nationwide. It was developed in an attempt to support those families who have difficulty accessing health and preschool services, and are suspicious of professional involvement. These families may sometimes find the flexible, informal, non–statutory relationship which a befriender can offer is a much more acceptable way of receiving support. Volunteers are trained, and then given ongoing supervision by the paid Homestart co-ordinator, while they befriend up to three local families. The volunteers visit regularly, aim to establish a supportive relationship with the mother, and then help her promote her child's development and engage with local services and resources. Local Homestart schemes may also offer additional activities, such as mothers' groups, outings, or playgroups.

Homestart schemes have been the subject of a number of external evaluations, none of which have involved a control group. One, which looked at the first Homestart scheme, found that the service had a very beneficial effect for a proportion of the families involved.[82] The majority of referrals came from social workers or health visitors, and 90% were of low income families, 40% were single parents, and 25% were on the child protection register. Many of the parents had histories of abuse. In the first 4 years there were 303 families referred, out of which 226 were matched with volunteers, and 156 became involved with the scheme for at least a few weeks, and many for much longer. A random sample of 30 was selected from the 156 engaged families. The degree of change in these families was investigated by asking involved professionals, volunteers and the families themselves. There was almost unanimous agreement that at least 50% of families had changed for the better, with health visitors being much more positive, identifying considerable change in 89% of families; 85% of the families themselves also said they had changed considerably. The volunteers were more cautious, identifying considerable change in only 47%; 4% of families said that they hadn't changed at all, whereas volunteers perceived no change in 13% of families. Social workers and health visitors, on the other hand, felt that all families involved had changed at least a little.

Newpin

The first Newpin centre was set up in South London in 1982. Several other Newpins have now been established, mainly in the South East of England. They work with families where the parents are depressed or distressed, and the children are at risk of abuse or have actually been abused. Referrals come from social workers, health visitors, and other agencies, self–referrals are also accepted. Referred families are assessed at home, and if suitable, may then be offered help from a befriender, attendance at the "drop–in", a client group, or individual counselling or therapy. Many members go on to train as volunteers after a period of time.

Apart from Newpin's founder, who had a background in health visiting, all Newpin centre co-ordinators were previously clients, who have completed a 2–year in–service training programme. A well designed evaluation compared outcomes for both new referrals and volunteers undergoing training, with a comparison group of mothers in similar circumstances who did not receive the Newpin service.[83] Unfortunately the study group of 40 families was small, and the study period was only 8 months. It was found that the mothers involved in Newpin were both exposed to serious current adversities, and had had very troubled childhoods, and that despite these problems, many of these mothers successfully trained as volunteers. However over the study period, 30% of the 40 mothers studied failed to sustain significant contact with Newpin. Those who were fully involved were extremely appreciative of the service and showed positive changes in self–esteem, sense of control over life, and psychiatric state. It appeared that mothers changed most during the second 6 months of their involvement with Newpin. Analysis of videotaped mother–child interactions before and after attending Newpin found a significant improvement in mothers' abilities to anticipate their children's needs, but otherwise no statistically significant improvements. For some mother–child pairs within the sample there were dramatic improvements, but for some pairs their relationship remained unsatisfactory. The small size of the study sample and the brevity of the evaluation period mean that the effectiveness of Newpin in altering mother–child relationships is best described as unproven, but many mothers feel greatly helped by the programme.

Community Mothers Programme

This well-evaluated programme in Ireland used non–professional volunteer community mothers to provide a child development programme to disadvantaged first time mothers in the first year of the child's life. Community mothers are women from the local community who are experienced parents, who have been trained, monitored and guided by paid family development nurses. Each family development nurse works in equal partnership with 15–20 community mothers. A randomised controlled trial compared mothers who received standard support from the public health nurse with those who had additional monthly visits from a community mother and found a number of positive outcomes. By the end of the programme, children in families visited by community mothers were more likely to have received all their immunisations, and be involved in cognitively stimulating activities with their mothers. Both children and mothers in these families had a significantly improved diet. Mothers also reported fewer feelings of fatigue and misery, and more positive feelings.[84] Since this evaluation was published, the programme has developed to include breastfeeding support, mother and toddler groups, and modified programmes for travellers.

As the above descriptions show, the voluntary sector can provide acceptable services to parents whom statutory services may find difficult to engage. But an actual improvement in the quality of parent–child relationships is not proven in the Newpin study, and not examined in Homestart evaluations. Despite this limitation, it is clear that services like this can meet an unmet need for family support. It is important, however, that the presence of the sorts of voluntary services described above should not encourage statutory services to withdraw. The voluntary sector and professional services need to maintain good communication and com-plementary working relationships for the interests of disadvantaged families to be best served.

Parenting education

Parenting education is discussed in a separate section because it is provided by all services and sectors involved with those aged 0–5. Parents usually learn about parenting in a variety of ways, including trial and error with their children, from family, community and media sources, and by reflecting on their own upbringing. Professionals and voluntary workers may provide education in parenting in several different ways. All of the services described above include some element of parent education, whether this is the provision of ad hoc advice at a parent's request, or work with parents on specific parenting issues. This section will focus on a different aspect of parenting education, involving formal parenting programmes which are generally used with groups.

Formal parenting programmes have been estimated as reaching some 28,000 parents (with children of all ages) per year, approximately 4% of those eligible.[85] The idea of learning about parenting in a group setting appears to be becoming more acceptable, though a proportion of families are likely to always remain unwilling to participate in this type of programme.

It has been suggested that parenting programmes are best delivered using a "lifecycle" approach.[86] This could include discussions of aspects of parenting as part of the curriculum for school age children, preparation for parenting for parents expecting their first child, and a range of programmes available to parents with children of different ages.

In reviewing the range of programmes available in a particular area, it is also important to consider particular local needs. Programmes may need to be tailored for different groups, for example, teenage parents, parents in prison, or parents with particular ethnic or religious identities.

The parenting programmes available in Britain today differ substantially in their precise content, theoretical underpinnings and style of delivery. They can be broadly divided according to their target group into programmes for those who want to do a "good–enough" job of parenting, programmes for parents whose children have "normal" behaviour problems, programmes for parents whose children have severe problems, and programmes for parents with multiple problems and low self–esteem. Despite these differences all parenting programmes tend to share a number of common purposes.[87] They encourage parents to:

- develop greater self–awareness;
- use effective discipline methods;
- improve parent–child communication;
- make family life more enjoyable;
- gain useful information about child development.

Pippin

This programme is designed to facilitate the transition to parenthood. It offers 17 group sessions to first time parents, starting in the fourth month of pregnancy and continuing until infants are 4–5 months old. The parent/s also receive a home visit after the child is born. The sessions are run by a highly trained facilitator who may be either a parent or a professional such as a midwife or health visitor. In a well-designed evaluation, 50 couples from a wide range of backgrounds were randomly selected to participate in nine pilot intervention groups, and 60 couples were designated as a control group. Parents who participated in the programme showed significantly more satisfaction and confidence as parents, greater clarity about their parenting role, an increase in nurturing child care attitudes, an increase in satisfaction with their couple relationship and their communication with their partner, an increase in self–esteem and psychological well–being, and a decrease in anxiety and vulnerability to depression. After 2–3 years, toddlers whose parents had participated in the programme were described as more calm and confident. More than 30 facilitators have now been trained, and groups have been run in different parts of the country.[88]

Parent Link

Parent Link groups are provided by Parent Network, in more than 30 local areas. The groups are intended for parents who want to be "good enough" at the job. Each course covers a number of topics with information provided in a small booklet at the end of each session. Many groups continue to meet without the facilitator when the course is finished. An uncontrolled independent evaluation found that 93% of parents felt more confident after attending a Parent Link group, 72% felt their children's behaviour had improved, and 95% of parents felt that they had gained new skills.[89]

Positive parenting

This programme has been specifically developed for parents of young children with difficult behaviour within the "normal" range. It involves eight group sessions and two group follow–ups, training parents in specific behaviour management skills. A controlled study comparing the effectiveness of training parents in these groups, in home visits, and by telephone contact found little difference between the three groups, with all methods producing an improvement in behaviour, which persisted for 12–18 months according to independent assessors. After this the maintenance of improvements declined, most markedly for the telephone method.[90]

ABC of behaviour

This programme is also intended for parents whose children have difficult behaviour within the "normal" range. It consists of six workshops, and parents are given an accompanying booklet. The programme has been

145

evaluated in five nursery schools, comparing 16 mother–child pairs where the mother attended the groups with 16 mother–child pairs who did not. Questionnaires were used before and after the programme to assess the level of behaviour problems, the mother's knowledge of behaviour strategies, and the mother's sense of self–esteem and competence. Teachers also assessed the child's behaviour in school. The author reported cautious optimism that the number of behaviour difficulties reported by both the mother and the teacher decreased, and the mother's knowledge of behavioural strategies increased.[91]

Handling children's behaviour

This programme of ten 2-hourly sessions is used widely in the West Midlands in day care settings and family centres. It is designed to help parents whose children have behaviour problems in the "normal" range. It has been evaluated by comparing delivery of the programme to eight mothers individually, nine mothers in a group, and 11 "control" mothers who attended a discussion group and received written information on child development, using validated questionnaires. Mothers receiving the programme individually and mothers in the group programme both showed significant improvements in their attitudes towards their children. Mothers seen individually showed a significant increase in their knowledge of behavioural principles, and those in the group programme reported raised self–esteem and reduction in the numbers of behaviour problems in their children. There was no change in the control group.

The following are examples of parenting programmes with families of young children run by specialised child mental health services.

The Parents and Children Series

This programme is intended to help parents whose children have severe behaviour problems. The programme is intended for older preschool or primary school children. It uses a model of parent management training developed in America by Patterson,[92] and Forehand and MacMahon,[93] and further refined by Webster–Stratton et al.[94] Groups of seven to ten families attend twelve 2-hour groups, without their children, and are trained in the principles of behaviour management using videotaped vignettes as the basis of group discussion. American outcome studies show that group work is as effective as one–to–one instruction, but at a quarter of the cost of therapist time. Initial research with British groups of families has found a low drop-out rate, and that all groups improved on conduct disorder scores, with individuals with severe conduct disorder problems improving markedly, and 1-year follow–up showed persistence of the improvements with no loss. A randomised controlled trial is under way on tier 2 and 3 services.

Mellow parenting

This intensive parenting day programme for families facing multiple adversities is provided in a London teaching hospital and some family centres in Scotland. Parents are provided with an intensive group based programme including psychotherapy and both direct and video work with parents. The programme is provided by a specially trained multidisciplinary team of social workers, psychologists, psychiatrists, occupational therapists, nurses, and creche workers. A pilot study of the effects of the programmes on 21 mothers found that there was a considerable positive change in interaction and child–centredness. Negative interaction dropped to one-quarter of the pregroup level, 10 of the 12 children on the Child Protection Register had their names removed. A larger controlled study with longer-term follow–up is currently under way.[95]

Summary

This review of key concepts, risk and protective factors, and national and local initiatives likely to improve young children's mental health presents a cautiously optimistic picture. We know what needs to be done, we have a framework for analysing the range of services addressing children's mental health problems, and some effective initiatives are already in place. It is clear that efforts to improve children's mental health need to be planned and evaluated in a coherent strategy across and between agencies, and be available to families over time, rather than as single interventions. In addition there is a need for a baseline level of universal services with further resources for high risk groups or areas of deprivation. The recent government funding of the National Parenting Institute, Parentline, an expanded role for health visitors, the Sure Start programme, and increased benefits for children and families are all encouraging developments. However the rhetoric of collaboration, innovation and development rings hollow when services at local level are faced with funding cuts and closures. Preserving adequate funding for prevention and early intervention in the face of demands from acute services remains problematical. But the provision of family support services, parent education, help for mothers with postnatal depression, and accessible advice for families where children have emotional and behavioural problems all have the potential to improve young children's mental health and save money at a later date. Choosing to prioritise the needs of young children both improves the quality of life for those children and their families in the short term, and also contributes to the well–being of society in the future.

1 Rutter M, Smith DJ. *Psychosocial Disorders in Young People: time trends and their causes.* Chichester: Wiley, 1995

2 Caspi A, Moffit TE, Newman DL, *et al.* Behavioral observations at three years predict adult psychiatric disorders: longitudinal evidence from a birth cohort. *Archives of General Psychiatry* 1996;**53**:1033–9

3 NHS Health Advisory Service. *Child and Adolescent Mental Health Services: together we stand.* London: HMSO, 1995

4 Winnicott DW. *The Maturational Process and the Facilitative Environment.* New York: International Universities Press, 1965

5 Goodman R, Scott S. *Child Psychiatry.* Oxford: Blackwell, 1997

6 Richman N, Stevenson J, Graham PJ. *Preschool to School: a behavioural study.* London: Academic Press, 1982

7 Earls F, Richman N. The prevalence of behaviour problems in 3–year-old children of West Indian born parents. *Journal of Child Psychology and Psychiatry* 1980;**21**:99–106

8 Campbell SB. Behaviour problems in preschool children: a review of recent research. *Journal of Child Psychology and Psychiatry* 1995;**36**:113–49

9 Strauss MA. *Beating the Devil out of Them: corporal punishment in American families.* New York: Lexington Books/Macmillan, 1994

10 Leach P. *The Physical Punishment of Children. Some input from recent research.* London: NSPCC Policy Practice Research Series, 1999

11 Hall DMB, ed. *Health for All Children.* Oxford: Oxford University Press, 1996

12 Rutter M. Psychosocial resilience and protective mechanisms. *American Journal of Orthopsychiatry* 1987;**57**:316–31

13 Office of Population Censuses and Surveys. *The Health of Our Children: decennial supplement.* Series DS no 11. London: HMSO, 1995

14 Office of Population Censuses and Surveys. *Living in Britain: results from the 1995 General Household Survey.* London: HMSO, 1997

15 Graham P. Prevention. In: Rutter M, Taylor E, Hersov L, eds. *Child and Adolescent Psychiatry: modern approaches.* Oxford: Blackwell, 1994

16 Blackburn C. *Poverty and Health: working with families.* Buckingham: Open University Press, 1991

17 Oppenheimer C, Harker L. *Poverty: the facts* London: Child Poverty Action Group, 1996

18 Hodes M. Refugee children. *British Medical Journal* 1998;**316**:794–5

19 Richman N. The effects of housing on pre–school children and their mothers. *Developmental Medicine and Child Neurology* 1974;**16**:53–8

20 Vostanis P, Grattan E, Cumella S. Mental health problems of homeless children and families: longitudinal study. *British Medical Journal* 1998;**316**:899–902

21 Carter EA, McGoldrick M. *The Family Lifecycle.* London: Gardner Press, 1980

22 Raphael–Leff J. *Psychological Processes of Childbearing.* London: Chapman & Hall, 1991

23 Polansky N, Gaudin J, Ammons P, *et al.* The psychological ecology of the neglectful mother. *Child Abuse and Neglect* 1985;**9**:265–75

24 Oakley A, Hickey D, Rajan L. Social support in pregnancy: does it have long–term effects? *Journal of Reproductive and Infant Psychology* 1996;**14**:7–22

25 Rutter M, Giller H, Hagell A. *Antisocial Behaviour by Young People.* Cambridge: Cambridge University Press, 1998

26 Rutter M, Cox A. Other family influences. In: Rutter M, Hersov L, eds. *Child & Adolescent Psychiatry: modern approaches.* Oxford: Blackwell, 1985

27 Hetherington EM, Cox M, Cox R. Long–term effects of divorce and remarriage on the adjustment of children. *Journal of the American Academy of Child and Adolescent Psychiatry* 1985;**24**:518–30

28 Monroe Blum H, Boyle MR, Offord R. Single parent families: child psychiatric disorder and school performance. *Journal of the American Academy of Child and Adolescent Psychiatry* 1988;**27**:214–19

29 Paterson CJ. Lesbian and gay parenthood. In: Bornstein MH, ed. *Handbook of Parenting*, vol 3. *Status and social conditions of parenting*. New Jersey: Lawrence Erlbaum, 1995

30 Lieberman A. *A Perspective on Infant Mental Health*. World Association for Infant Mental Health: The Signal, Jan–Mar, 1998

31 Mayes LC. Substance abuse and parenting. In: Bornstein MH, ed. *Handbook of Parenting*, vol 4. New Jersey: Lawrence Erlbaum, 1995

32 Lou HC, Hansen D, Nordenfoft M, *et al.* Prenatal stressors of human life affect fetal brain development. *Developmental Medicine and Child Neurology* 1994;**6**:826–32

33 Field T, Dandberg D, Quetel TA, *et al.* Effects of ultrasound feedback on pregnancy anxiety, fetal activity and neonatal outcome. *Obstetrics and Gynaecology* 1985;**66**:525–8

34 Rothberg AD, Lits B. Psychosocial support for maternal stress during pregnancy: effects on birthweight. *American Journal of Obstetrics and Gynecology* 1991;**65**:403–7

35 Villar J, Farnot U, Barros F, *et al.* A randomised trial of psychosocial support during high-risk pregnancies. *New England Journal of Medicine* 1992;**327**:1266–71

36 Maccoby EE, Martin JA. Socialisation in the context of the family. Parent–child interaction. In: Hetherington EM, ed. *Handbook of Child Psychology. Socialisation, personality and social development*, vol 4. New York: Wiley, 1983

37 Patterson GR, Reid JB, Dishion TJ. *A Social Learning Approach*, vol 4. *Antisocial boys*. Ontario: Castalia Publishing Company, 1992

38 Dornbusch SM, Ritter PL, Leiderman PH, *et al.* The relation of parenting style to adolescent school performance. *Child Development* 1987;**58**:1244 57

39 Lamborn S, Mounts NS, Steinberg L, *et al.* Patterns of competence and adjustment among adolescents from authoritative, authoritarian, indulgent and neglectful families. *Child Development* 1991;**62**:1049–65

40 Scarr S, McCartney K How people make their own environments: a theory of genotype–environment effects. *Annual Progress in Child Psychiatry and Child Development* 1984:98–118

41 Report of the Commission on Children and Violence. *Children and Violence*. London: Gulbenkian Foundation, 1995

42 Thompson EE. The short and long–term effects of corporal punishment on children. A meta–analytic review. *Psychological Bulletin* (in press)

43 Department of Health. Press Release 98/397, 23 September 1998

44 Home Office, Department of Health, Department of Education and Science, Welsh Office. *Working Together Under the Children's Act 1989: a guide to arrangements for interagency co–operation for the protection of children from abuse*. London: HMSO, 1991

45 Bannister A. Recognising abuse. In: Stainton–Rogers W, Hevey D, Ash E, eds. *Child Abuse and Neglect: facing the challenge*. London: BT Batsford, 1989

46 Garbarino J, Vondra J. Psychological maltreatment: issues and perspectives. In: Brassard M, Germain B, Hart S, eds. *Psychological Maltreatment of Children and Youth*. New York: Pergamon, 1987

47 Kaufman J, Zigler E. Do abused children become abusive parents? *American Journal of Orthopsychiatry* 1987;**57**:186–91

48 Quinton D, Rutter M. Family pathology and child psychiatric disorder: a four year prospective study. In: Nicol AR, ed. *Longitudinal Studies in Child Psychology and Psychiatry*. Chichester: Wiley, 1985

49 Cox JL, Holden JM, Sagorsky R. Detection of postnatal depression: development of the 10 item Edinburgh Postnatal Depression Scale. *British Journal of Psychiatry* 1987;**150**:782–6

50 Appleby L, Warner R, Whitton A, *et al.* A controlled study of fluoxetine and cognitive–behavioural counselling in the treatment of postnatal depression. *British Medical Journal* 1997;**314**:932–6

51 Clulow C, ed. *Partners Becoming Parents*. London: Sheldon Press, 1996

52 Scarr S, Eisenberg M. Child care research: issues, perspectives and results. *Annual Review of Psychology* 1993;**44**:613–44

53 Lamb ME, Sternberg KJ, Prodromis M. Non–maternal care and the security of infant–mother attachment: a re–analysis of the data. *Infant Behaviour and Development* 1992;**15**:71–83

54 Triseliotis J, Hill M. Contrasting adoption, foster care and residential rearing. In: Brodzinsky DM, Schechter MD, eds. *The Psychology of Adoption*. New York: Oxford University Press, 1990

55 Triseliotis J, Russell J. *Hard to Place: the outcome of late adoptions and residential care*. London: Heinemann, 1984

56 Hersov L. Adoption. In: Rutter M, Hersov L, Taylor E, eds. *Child and Adolescent Psychiatry: modern approaches*. Oxford: Blackwell, 1994

57 Hindley P. Psychiatric aspects of hearing impairments. *Journal of Child Psychology and Psychiatry* 1997;**38**:101–17

58 Baker L, Cantwell DP. Psychiatric disorder in children with different types of communication disorder. *Journal of Communication Disorders* 1982;**15**:113–26

59 Bowlby J. *Attachment and Loss*, vol 1. *Attachment*. New York: Basic Books, 1969

60 Bowlby J. *Attachment and Loss*, vol 2. *Separation: anger and anxiety*. New York: Basic Books, 1973

61 Bowlby J. *Attachment and Loss*, vol 3. *Loss, sadness and depression*. New York: Basic Books, 1980

62 Spieker SJ, Booth CL. Maternal antecedents of attachment quality. In: Belsky J, Nezworski T, eds. *Clinical Implications of Attachment*. New Jersey: Erlbaum, 1988

63 DeMulder EK, Radke–Yarrow M. Attachment with affectively ill and well mothers: concurrent behavioural correlates. *Development and Psychopathology* 1991;**3**:227–42

64 Cichetti D, Barnett D. Attachment organisation in maltreated preschoolers. *Development and Psychology* 1991;**3**:397–411

65 Lyons–Ruth K, Alpen L, Repacholi B. Disorganised infant classification and maternal psychosocial problems as predictors of hostile–aggressive behaviour in the preschool classroom. *Child Development* 1993;**64**:572–85

66 American Psychiatric Association. *DSM–IV: diagnostic and statistical manual of mental disorders*, 4th edn. Washington DC: American Psychiatric Association, 1994

67 World Health Organisation. *The ICD–10 Classification of Mental and Behavioural Disorders: clinical descriptions and diagnostic guidelines*. Geneva: World Health Organisation, 1992

68 Hodges J, Tizard B. Social and family relationships of ex–institutional adolescents. *Journal of Child Psychology, Psychiatry and Allied Disciplines* 1989;**30**: 77–97

69 Scarr S, Weinberg RA. The early childhood enterprise, care and education of the young. *American Psychologist* 1986;**41**:1140–6

70 Billingham K, Hall D. Turbulent future for school nursing and health visiting. *British Medical Journal* 1998;**316**:406–7

71 Hayden A. A GP based child and adolescent mental health service. *Young Minds* 1997;**30**:12–13

72 Holden JM, Sagovsky R, Cox JL. Counselling in a general practice setting: controlled study of health visitor intervention in treatment of postnatal depression. *British Medical Journal* 1989;**298**:223–6

73 Barker WE, Anderson RA, Chalmers C. *Health Trends over Time and Major Outcomes of the Child Development Programme*. Belfast: Eastern Health and Social Services Board, Bristol ECDU, 1994

74 Davis H, Spurr D, Cox A, *et al*. A descriptive evaluation of a community child health mental health service. *Clinical Child Psychology and Psychiatry* 1997;**2**:221–8

75 Bromley by Bow Centre. *Annual Review 1996–1997*. London: The Centre, 1997

76 Aldgate J, Tunstill J. *Making Sense of Section 17. Implementing services for children in need within the 1989 Children Act*. London: HMSO, 1995

77 Gibbons J, Thorpe S, Wilkinson P. *Family Support and Prevention*. London: National Institute for Social Work, HMSO, 1990

78 Makins V. *Not Just a Nursery . . . multi–agency early years centres in action*. London: National Childrens Bureau, 1997

79 Schweinhart L, Barnes H, Weikart D. *The High Scope Perry pre-school study through age 27.* Michigan: High Scope Press, 1993

80 Lazar I, Darlington R. Lasting effects of early education. *Monograph of Society for Research in Child Development* 1982;**47**:2–3

81 O'Flaherty J. *Highlight 131 High Scope.* London: National Children's Bureau, 1995

82 Van der Eyken W. *Homestart: a four year evaluation.* Leicester: Home–Start Consultancy, 1990

83 Cox AD, Pound A, Puckering C, *et al.* Evaluation of a home visiting and befriending scheme: Newpin. *Journal of the Royal Society of Medicine* 1991;**84**:217–20

84 Johnson Z, Howell F, Molloy B. Community Mothers Programme: randomised controlled trial of non–professional intervention in parenting. *British Medical Journal* 1993;**306**: 1449–52

85 Smith C. *Developing Parenting Programmes.* London: National Children's Bureau, 1997

86 Pugh G, De'ath E, Smith C. *Confident Parents, Confident Children: policy and practice in parent education and support.* London: National Children's Bureau, 1994

87 Smith C, Pugh G. *Learning to be a Parent: a survey of group–based parenting programmes.* London: Family Policy Studies Centre, 1996

88 Parr MA. *Support for Couples in the Transition to Parenthood.* University of East London, 1996 (unpublished PhD thesis)

89 David H, Hester P. *An Independent Evaluation of Parent–link, A Parenting Education Programme Developed by Parent Network Academic Unit of Child and Adolescent Psychiatry and Psychology.* London: United Medical and Dental Schools, 1997

90 Sutton C. Parent training by telephone: a partial replication. *Behavioural Psychotherapy* 1995;**20**:115–39

91 Hinton S. *A Study of Behaviour Management Workshops for Parents of Nursery School Children.* A report submitted for an associateship at the Institute of Education, University of London, 1987

92 Patterson GR. *Families: applications of social learning to family life,* revised edn. Champaign, Illinois: Research Press, 1975

93 Forehand R, MacMahon RJ. *Helping the Non–compliant Child: a clinician's guide to effective parent training.* New York: Guildford Press, 1981

94 Webster Stratton C, Kolpacoff M, Hollinsworth T. The long–term effectiveness of three cost–effective training programs for families with conduct problem children. *Journal of Consulting and Clinical Psychology* 1989;**57**:550 3

95 Puckering C, Rogers J, Mills M, *et al.* Process and evaluation of a group intervention for mothers with parenting difficulties. *Child Abuse Review* 1994;**3**:299–310

Chapter 8 - Fetal origins of adult disease

The rewards of good health care in childhood, especially health promotion and preventative interventions, are unique because the benefits may last a lifetime and maybe passed onto future generations.

(House of Commons Health Committee, 1997)

A number of studies have found that not only do unfavourable socio-economic conditions in childhood and during fetal development affect health in childhood but they also predispose to increased risk of disease in adulthood. The research that points to this link began as a means of explaining the differences in rates of heart disease that could not be explained by known risk factors such as obesity and smoking. There was evidence that in areas where there were high rates of death from cardiovascular disease, there used to be high infant death rates. It was therefore considered that factors with an adverse effect on infant health may have adverse effects in adult life. This means that protecting the health of children in the early years becomes even more crucial.

The programming theory of health

Recent findings suggest that some answers may lie in influences which act in fetal and infant life and permanently set structures and metabolic processes, so-called "programming".[1] The steep rise in coronary heart disease (CHD) in Britain during this century has been associated with rising prosperity, but the poorest people in the least affluent places have the highest rates of CHD. These differences in CHD are a major contributor to the socio-economic inequalities of life expectancy in Britain. The geographical distribution of neonatal mortality (deaths before 1 month of age) in England and Wales in the early years of this century closely resembled the distribution of death rates from cardiovascular disease today (Figure 8.1).[2]

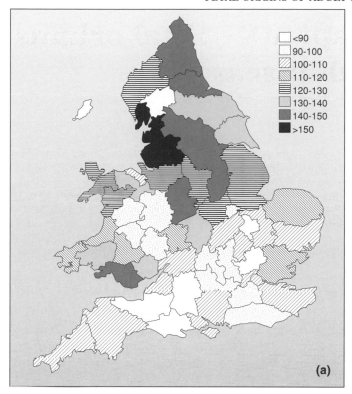

Fig 8.1 Similarity between the distribution of neonatal mortality and coronary heart disease mortality. (a) Infant mortality in England and Wales 1901–10. (Source: Local Government Board. *Forty Second Annual Report 1912 1913. Second report on infant and child mortality.* London: HMSO, 1913)

At that time most neonatal deaths were attributed to low birthweight. One interpretation of this geographical association is that harmful influences which act in fetal life, and slow fetal growth, permanently set or "programme" the body's structure and function in ways which are linked to cardiovascular disease.

The large geographical and social class differences in fetal and infant growth which existed in Britain when today's generation of middle-aged and elderly people were born, were reflected in the wide range of infant mortality. In 1921–25 infant mortality ranged from 44 deaths per 1000 births in rural West Sussex to 114 per 1000 births in Burnley. The highest rates were generally in northern counties where large manufacturing towns had grown up around the coal seams, and in impoverished rural areas such as north Wales. They were lowest in counties in the south and east, which have the best agricultural land and are historically the wealthiest. A series of

153

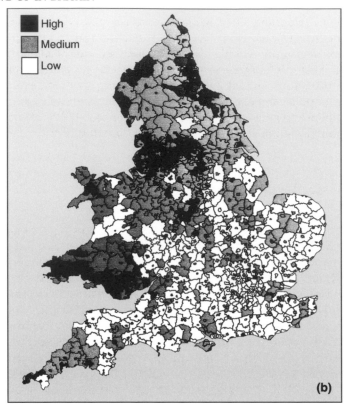

High
Medium
Low

(b)

Fig 8.1 Similarity between the distribution of neonatal mortality and coronary heart disease mortality. (b) Coronary heart disease mortality in England and Wales: 1968–70. (Source: Gardner MJ, Winter PD, Barker DJP. *Atlas of Mortality from Selected Diseases in England and Wales. 1968–1978.* Chichester: John Wiley, 1984. Reproduced with permission.)

government inquiries on child and maternal mortality from 1910 onwards, prompted by revelations of the poor physique of military recruits, showed how these differences in infant mortality were related to differences in the nutrition and health of young women, infant feeding, housing, and overcrowding.[3] Undernutrition of the fetus is an obvious possible harmful influence and numerous studies in animals have shown that fetal undernutrition permanently programmes physiology and metabolism.[4, 5]

In fetal life the tissues and organs of the body go through what are called "critical" periods of development which may coincide with periods of rapid cell division. "Programming" describes the process whereby a stimulus causing a positive or negative response at a critical period of development has lasting effects. Rickets has for a long while served as a demonstration that undernutrition at a critical stage of early life leads to persisting changes in the body's structure. Only recently have we realised that some of the persisting effects of early undernutrition become translated into pathology, and thereby determine chronic disease, including cardiovascular disease, in later life.[1, 5] That this has gone unremarked for so long is perhaps surprising, given the numerous animal experiments showing that undernutrition *in utero* leads to persisting changes in blood pressure, cholesterol metabolism, insulin response to glucose, and a range of other metabolic, endocrine and immune functions known to be important in human disease.[5, 6]

Undernutrition *in utero*

The human fetus adapts to undernutrition by metabolic changes, redistribution of blood flow, and changes in the production of fetal and placental hormones which control growth.[7] Its immediate response to undernutrition is catabolism; it consumes its own substrates to provide energy.[8] More prolonged undernutrition leads to a slowing in growth. This enhances the fetus' ability to survive by reducing the use of substrates and lowering the metabolic rate. Slowing of growth in late gestation leads to disproportion in organ size, because organs and tissues that are growing rapidly at the time are affected the most. Undernutrition in late gestation may, for example, lead to reduced growth of the kidney, which develops rapidly at that time. Reduced replication of kidney cells in late gestation will permanently reduce cell numbers, because after birth there seems to be no capacity for renal cell division to "catch up".

Animal studies show that a variety of different patterns of fetal growth result in similar birth size. A fetus that grows slowly throughout gestation may have the same size at birth as a fetus whose growth was arrested for a period and then "caught up". Different patterns of fetal growth will have different effects on the relative size of different organs at birth, even though overall body size may be the same. Animal studies show that blood pressure and metabolism can be permanently changed by levels of undernutrition that do not influence growth. Preliminary observations point to similar effects in humans. Such findings emphasise the severe limitation of birthweight as a summary of fetal nutritional experience.

While slowing its rate of growth the fetus may protect tissues that are important for immediate survival, the brain especially. One way in which the brain can be protected is by redistribution of blood flow to favour it.[9] This adaptation is known to occur in many mammals but in humans it has exaggerated costs for tissues other than the brain, notably the liver and other abdominal viscera, because of the large size of the human brain. Metabolic fetal adaptations may result in the baby sacrificing muscle growth and being born thin.

155

It is becoming increasingly clear that nutrition has profound effects on fetal hormones, and on the hormonal and metabolic interactions between the fetus, placenta and mother on whose co-ordination fetal growth depends.[8] Fetal insulin and the insulin-like growth factors (IGFs) are thought to have a central role in the regulation of growth and respond rapidly to changes in fetal nutrition. If a mother decreases her food intake, fetal insulin, IGF and glucose concentrations fall, possibly through the effect of decreased maternal IGF. This leads to reduced transfer of amino acids and glucose from mother to fetus, and ultimately to reduced rates of fetal growth.[10] In late gestation and after birth the fetus' growth hormone and IGF axis take over from insulin, a central role in driving linear growth. Whereas undernutrition leads to a fall in the concentrations of hormones that control fetal growth it leads to a rise in cortisol, whose main effects are on cell differentiation.[7] One current line of research aims to determine whether the fetus' hormonal adaptations to undernutrition tend, like many other fetal adaptations, to persist after birth and exert lifelong effects on homeostasis and hence on the occurrence of disease. Undernutrition during pregnancy can affect both placental size and body size of the baby at birth, and recent research has shown that, in turn, they can influence health.

Cardiovascular disease

Cardiovascular disease and body size at birth

The early epidemiological studies on the intra-uterine origins of coronary heart disease and stroke were based on the simple strategy of examining men and women in middle and late life whose body measurements were recorded at birth. The birth records on which these studies were based came to light as a result of the Medical Research Council's systematic search of the archives and records offices of Britain – a search that led to the discovery of three important groups of records in Hertfordshire, Preston, and Sheffield. The Hertfordshire records were maintained by health visitors and include measurements of growth in infancy as well as birthweight. In Preston and Sheffield detailed obstetric records documented body proportions at birth.

Sixteen thousand men and women born in Hertfordshire from 1911 to 1930 have now been traced from birth to the present day. Death rates from CHD fall twofold between those at the lower and upper ends of the birthweight distribution (Table 8.1).

A study in Sheffield showed that it was people who were small at birth because they failed to grow, rather than because they were born early, who were at increased risk of disease.[11] The association between low birthweight and CHD has been confirmed in studies of men in Uppsala, Sweden[12] and

Table 8.1   Death rates from coronary heart disease among 15,726 men and women according to birthweight

Birthweight pounds*	Standardised mortality ratio	Deaths (no.)
≤ 5.5 (2.50)	100	57
– 6.5 (2.95)	81	137
– 7.5 (3.41)	80	298
– 8.5 (3.86)	74	289
– 9.5 (4.31)	55	103
> 9.5 (4.31)	65	57
Total	74	941

* Figures in parentheses are kilograms.
(This table was first published in the BMJ (Osmond C, Barker DJP, Winter PD *et al.* Early growth and death from cardiovascular disease in women. *British Medical Journal* 1993;**307**:1519–24) and is reproduced by permission of the BMJ)

Caerphilly, Wales[13] and among 80,000 women in the USA who took part in the American nurses study.[14] An association between low birthweight and prevalent CHD has also recently been shown in a study in South India.[15]

Cardiovascular disease and body proportions at birth

The Hertfordshire records and the American nurses and Caerphilly studies did not include measurements of body size at birth other than weight. The weight of a newborn baby without a measure of its length is as crude a summary of its physique as is the weight of a child or adult without a measure of height. The addition of birth length allows a thin baby to be distinguished from a stunted baby with the same birthweight. With the addition of head circumference the baby whose body is small in relation to its head, which may be a result of "brain-sparing" redistribution of blood flow, can also be distinguished. Thinness, stunting and a low birthweight in relation to head size are the result of differing fetal adaptations to undernutrition, and other influences, and they have different consequences, both immediately and in the long term.

In Sheffield death rates for CHD were higher in men who were stunted at birth.[16] The mortality ratio for CHD in men who were 47 cm or less in length was 138 compared with 98 in the remainder.[16] Similarly CHD in South India was associated with stunting.[15] Thinness at birth, as measured by a low ponderal index (birthweight/length),[11] is also associated with CHD. Table 8.2 shows findings among men born in Helsinki, Finland from 1924 to 1933. Death rates for CHD were related to low birthweight.[17] There was, however, a much stronger association with thinness at birth to CHD. Men who were thin at birth, measured by a low ponderal index (birthweight/length)[11] had death rates that were twice those of men who had a high ponderal index (Table 8.3).

157

Table 8.2   Hazard ratios for coronary heart disease in 3641 Finnish men born during 1924–33 according to birthweight

Birthweight kg*	Men (no.)	Hazard ratios	Deaths (no.)
≤ 2.5 (5.5)	145	1.13	11
– 3.0 (6.6)	557	1.23	44
– 3.5 (7.7)	1328	1.46	133
– 4.0 (8.8)	1165	1.11	88
> 4.0 (8.8)	446	1.00	30

P value for trend adjusted for gestation = 0.05
* Figures in parentheses are pounds.
(This table was first published in the BMJ (Forsen T, Eriksson JG, Tuomilehto J et al. Mother's weight in pregnancy and coronary heart disease in a cohort of Finnish men: follow-up study. British Medical Journal 1997;**315**:837–40) and is reproduced by permission of the BMJ)

Trends in stroke, which have only been reported among men in Sheffield, are different to those in CHD. While stroke has a similar association with birthweight it is not related to stunting or thinness. Rather, high rates are associated with a low ratio of birthweight to head circumference. This finding has recently been confirmed in Finland (unpublished).

Cardiovascular disease and infant growth

Information routinely recorded in Hertfordshire included the infant's weight at aged 1 year. In men, failure of weight gain during the first year of life predicted CHD and stroke independently of birthweight.[16] Among men who weighed 8.0 kg or less at age 1 year, rates of CHD were twice those among men who weighed 12.2 kg or more. The highest rates of the disease among men were in those who had both low birthweight and low weight at age 1 year. By contrast, the highest rates among women were in those who had low birthweight but whose weight "caught up" before aged 1 year. The

Table 8.3   Hazard ratios by thinness at birth (ponderal index) for coronary heart disease in 3641 Finnish men born during 1924–33

Ponderal index at birth (kg/m³)	Men (no.)	Hazard ratios	Deaths (no.)
≤25	724	2.07	82
- 27	1099	1.75	106
- 29	1081	1.33	80
>29	722	1.00	41

P value for trend adjusted for gestation < 0.0001
(This table was first published in the BMJ (Barker DJP, Osmond C, Simmonds SJ et al. The relation of small head circumference and thinness at birth to death from cardiovascular disease in adult life. British Medical Journal 1993;**306**:422–6) and is reproduced by permission of the BMJ)

reasons for this are unknown, although it may reflect sex differences in the endocrine control of infant growth. Growth during infancy can be regarded as a postnatal continuation of the fetal phase of growth, which is controlled by insulin and insulin-like growth factor I and continues until growth hormone takes over around the age of 1 year.[18]

Confounding effects of childhood circumstances

These findings suggest that influences linked to fetal and infant growth have an important effect on the risk of CHD and stroke. People whose growth was impaired *in utero* and during infancy are likely to continue to be exposed to an adverse environment in childhood and adult life, although some have argued that it is this later environment that produces the effects attributed to "programming".[19–22] There is strong evidence against this. In three of the studies on the association between birthweight and CHD, data on lifestyle factors including smoking, employment, alcohol consumption, and exercise were collected[12] and the associations between birthweight and CHD were little changed by allowing for these lifestyle factors (Figure 8.2).

Bartley *et al.* concluded that the implications of low birthweight for future health will be better understood if biological and socio-economic trajectories are investigated in combination. Studies which document experiences right through from birth to adulthood are required if the elucidation of mechanisms linking early life experience and disease in adulthood is to be taken forward.[23]

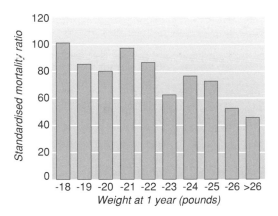

Fig 8.2 Death rates from coronary heart disease in 10,141 men according to weight at 1 year. (This figure was first published in the BMJ (Osmond C, Barker DJP, Winter PD *et al.* Early growth and death from cardiovascular disease in women. *British Medical Journal* 1993;**307**:1519–24) and is reproduced by permission of the BMJ)

Table 8.4   Prevalence of non-insulin dependent diabetes mellitus (NIDDM) and impaired glucose tolerance in men aged 59–70 years

Birthweight pounds*	Men (no.)	% with impaired glucose tolerance or NIDDM (plasma glucose ≤7.8 mmol/l)	Odds ratio adjusted for body mass index (95% confidence interval)
≤5.5 (2.50)	20	40	6.6 (1.5 to 28)
– 6.5 (2.95)	47	34	4.8 (1.3–17)
– 7.5 (3.41)	104	31	4.6 (1.4–16)
– 8.5 (3.86)	117	22	2.6 (0.8–8.9)
– 9.5 (4.31)	54	13	1.4 (0.3–5.6)
> 9.5 (4.31)	28	14	1.0
Total	370	25	

* Figures in parentheses are kilograms.
(This table was first published in the BMJ (Hales CN, Barker DJP, Clark PMS *et al*. Fetal and infant growth and impaired glucose tolerance at age 64. *British Medical Journal* 1991;**303**:1019–22) and is reproduced by permission of the BMJ)

In studies exploring the mechanisms underlying these associations, the trends in CHD with birthweight have been found to be paralleled by similar trends in two of its major risk factors – hypertension and non-insulin dependent diabetes mellitus.[24, 25] Table 8.4 illustrates the size of these trends.

The associations between small size at birth and hypertension and non-insulin dependent diabetes are again independent of social class, cigarette smoking, and alcohol consumption. Influences in adult life, however, add to the effects of the intra-uterine environment. For example, the prevalence of impaired glucose tolerance is highest in people who had low birthweight but became obese as adults.

Hypertension

Hypertension and body size at birth

Associations between low birthweight and raised blood pressure in childhood and adult life, such as those in a sample of the Hertfordshire cohort shown in Table 8.5, have been extensively demonstrated around the world.

Figure 8.3 shows the results of a systematic review of published papers describing the association between birthweight and blood pressure – the review is based on 34 studies of more than 66,000 people of all ages in many countries.[24] Each point on the figure, with its confidence interval, represents a study population and the populations are ordered by their ages. The horizontal position of each population describes the change in blood pressure that was associated with an increase in 1 kg birthweight. In almost all the studies an increase in birthweight was associated with a fall in blood

Table 8.5 Mean systolic blood pressure in men and women aged 60–71 years according to birthweight

Birthweight pounds*	Systolic blood pressure adjusted for sex (mmHg)	Subjects (no.)
– 5.5 (2.50)	168	54
– 6.5 (2.95)	165	174
– 7.5 (3.41)	165	403
– 8.5 (3.86)	164	342
– 9.5 (4.31)	160	183
>9.5 (4.31)	163	72
All	164	1228
Standard deviation	25	

* Figures in parentheses are kilograms.
(This table was first published in the BMJ (Law CM, de Swiet M, Osmond C *et al*. Initiation of hypertension *in utero* and its amplification throughout life. *British Medical Journal* 1993;**306**:24–7) and is reproduced by permission of the BMJ)

pressure, and there was no exception to this in the studies of adults which now total nearly 8000 men and women. The associations are less consistent in adolescence, presumably because the tracking of blood pressure from childhood through adult life is perturbed by the adolescent growth spurt. The associations between birthweight and blood pressure are not confounded by socio-economic conditions at the time of birth or in adult life.[26] Although the differences in mean systolic pressure are small by clinical standards, their public health implications are significant. Available data suggest that lowering the mean systolic pressure in a population by 10 mmHg would correspond to a 30% reduction in total attributable mortality.[27]

Similarly to CHD and stroke, the association between low birthweight and raised blood pressure depends on babies who were small for dates, after reduced fetal growth, rather than on babies who were born preterm.[12]

In the various studies of adults, alcohol consumption and higher body mass have been associated with raised blood pressure, although the associations between birthweight and blood pressure were independent of them. Nevertheless body mass remains an important influence on blood pressure and the highest pressures are found in people who were small at birth but become overweight as adults.[12]

As has already been emphasised birthweight is a crude indicator of fetal nutrition and growth because it fails to distinguish stunting, thinness and low birthweight in relation to head size and because levels of undernutrition which are too slight to influence growth may nevertheless programme metabolism. In contrast to the associations between birth size and CHD however, those between low birthweight and raised blood pressure are generally as strong as those between thinness or stunting and raised blood pressure.[28, 29]

161

Hypertension and placental size

Table 8.6 shows the systolic pressure of a group of men and women who were born, at term, in Sharoe Green Hospital in Preston, 50 years ago.

The subjects are grouped according to their birthweights and placental weights. Consistent with findings in other studies, systolic pressure falls between subjects with low and high birthweight. In addition, however, there is an increase in blood pressure with increasing placental weight. Subjects with a mean systolic pressure of 150 mmHg or more, a level sometimes used to define hypertension in clinical practice, comprise a group who as babies were relatively small in relation to the size of their placentas.

Hypertension and fetal undernutrition

Several lines of evidence support the thesis that it is poor delivery of nutrients and oxygen which programmes raised blood pressure in humans.

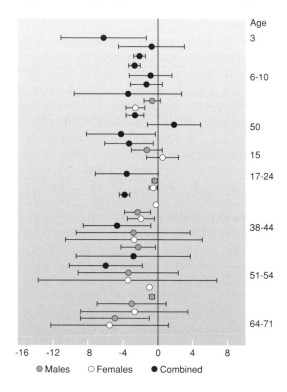

Fig 8.3 Difference in systolic pressure (mmHg) per kg increase in birthweight (adjusted for weight in children and body mass index in adults). (Source: Law CM, Shield AW. Is blood pressure inversely related to birthweight? The strength of evidence from a systematic review of the literature. *Journal of Hypertension* 1996;**14**:935–41)

Table 8.6   Mean systolic blood pressure (mmHg) of men and women aged 50, born after 38 completed weeks of gestation, according to placental weight and birthweight

Birthweight pounds*	Placental weight†				All
	≤ 1.0 lb (454g)	− 1.25 lb (568g)	− 1.5 lb (681g)	>1.5 lb (681g)	
− 6.5 (2.9)	149 (24)	152 (46)	151 (18)	167 (6)	152 (94)
− 7.5 (3.4)	139 (16)	148 (63)	146 (35)	159 (23)	148 (137)
>7.5 (3.4)	131 (3)	143 (23)	148 (30)	153 (40)	149 (96)
Total	144 (43)	148 (132)	148 (83)	156 (69)	149‡ (327)

* Figures in parentheses are kilograms.
† Figures in parentheses are numbers of subjects.
‡ SD = 20.4.
(This table was first published in the BMJ (Barker DJP, Bull AR, Osmond C *et al.* Fetal and placental size and risk of hypertension in adult life. *British Medical Journal* 1990;**301**:259–62) and is reproduced by permission of the BMJ)

First, experimental undernutrition of pregnant animals is known to cause lifelong elevation in the blood pressure of the offspring.[30, 31] In humans, a mother's fatness, weight gain in pregnancy and diet may all be related to the offspring's blood pressure, whereas other influences on fetal growth, including maternal height, parity and cigarette smoking are unrelated to the offspring's blood pressure, other than in small preterm babies.[32, 33] In Jamaica, children whose mothers had thin triceps skinfolds in early pregnancy and low weight gain during pregnancy had raised blood pressure.[34] There were similar findings in a group of children in Birmingham.[35] In the Gambia low pregnancy weight gain was associated with higher blood pressure in childhood.[36] In Aberdeen the blood pressures of middle-aged men and women were found to be related to their mother's intakes of carbohydrate and protein during pregnancy.[37]

Mechanisms

A number of possible mechanisms linking reduced fetal growth and raised blood pressure are currently being investigated. The rise of blood pressure during childhood is closely related to the rate of growth, and is accelerated by the adolescent growth spurt. This has led to the suggestion that essential hypertension is a disorder of growth.[38]

Non-insulin dependent diabetes (NIDD)

Insulin has a central role in fetal growth, and disorders of glucose and insulin metabolism are an obvious possible link between early growth and

163

cardiovascular disease. Although obesity and a sedentary lifestyle are known to be important in the development of non-insulin dependent diabetes, they seem to lead to the disease only in predisposed individuals. Family and twin studies have suggested that the predisposition is familial, but the nature of this predisposition is unknown. The disease tends to be transmitted through the mother's side of the family.

NIDD and body size at birth

A number of studies have confirmed the association between birthweight, impaired glucose tolerance and non-insulin dependent diabetes first reported in Hertfordshire.[39-44] Studies in Preston and Uppsala, Sweden, where detailed birth measurements were available, found that thinness at birth was more strongly related than birthweight to impaired glucose tolerance and non-insulin dependent diabetes.[40,41] Table 8.7 shows that in Uppsala the prevalence of diabetes was three times higher among men in the lowest fifth of ponderal index at birth.

Among the Pima Indians in the USA a raised prevalence of NIDD was associated with both low birthweight and with birthweights over 4.5 kg.[44] The increased risk of NIDD among babies with high birthweights was associated with maternal diabetes in pregnancy, which is unusually common in this community.

The adverse effects of low birthweight and thinness at birth on glucose/insulin metabolism are already evident in childhood. Seven-year-old children in Salisbury who were thin at birth had raised plasma glucose concentrations after an oral load.[45] In a group of older British children those who had lower birthweights had raised plasma insulin concentrations, both fasting and after oral glucose.[46] This is consistent with the association between low birthweight and insulin resistance. Low birthweight or

Table 8.7 Prevalence of non-insulin dependent diabetes by ponderal index at birth among 60 year old men in Uppsala, Sweden

Ponderal index at birth (kg/m³)	Men (no.)	Prevalence of diabetes (%)
< 24.2	193	11.9
24.2 –	193	5.2
25.9 –	196	3.6
27.4 –	188	4.3
≥ 29.4	201	3.5
Total	971	5.7

P value for trend 0.001
(This table was first published in the BMJ (Lithell HO, McKeigue PM, Berglund L *et al.* Relation of size at birth to non-insulin dependent diabetes and insulin concentrations in men aged 50–60 years. *British Medical Journal* 1996;**312**:406–10) and is reproduced by permission of the BMJ)

stunting at birth have been found to be associated with reduced glucose tolerance among children in India and Jamaica. These findings in children provide further support for the hypothesis that NIDD originates from impaired development *in utero* and that the seeds of the disease in the next generation have not only been sown but are already apparent in today's children.

Mechanisms

The processes that link thinness at birth with insulin resistance in adult life are not known. Babies born at term with a low ponderal index have a reduced mid-arm circumference, which implies that they have a low muscle bulk as well as less subcutaneous fat. One possibility is that thinness at birth is associated with abnormalities in muscle structure and function which persist into adult life, interfering with insulin's ability to promote glucose uptake.[47] Another possibility is that insulin resistance represents persistence of a glucose-sparing metabolism adopted in fetal life in response to undernutrition. The undernourished fetus reduces its metabolic dependence on glucose and increases oxidation of other substrates, including amino acids and lactate. A third possibility is that persisting hormonal changes underlie the development of insulin resistance. Glucocorticoids, growth hormone and sex steroids are thought to play a major role in the evolution of the insulin resistance syndrome.[48]

Serum cholesterol and blood clotting

Studies in Sheffield show that the neonate that has a reduced abdominal circumference at birth, although within the normal range of birthweight, has persisting disturbances of cholesterol metabolism and blood coagulation which predispose to CHD.[49, 50] This is thought to reflect impaired growth of the liver, two of whose functions are regulation of cholesterol and blood clotting. The differences in serum total and low density lipoprotein cholesterol concentrations across the range of abdominal circumference are large, statistically equivalent to 30% differences in mortality caused by CHD (Table 8.8).

Chronic bronchitis and fetal growth

Much of the socio-economic and geographical inequality in death rates in Britain is the result of differences in the occurrence of cardiovascular disease and chronic airflow obstruction. Death rates from "chronic bronchitis" are highest in the cities and large towns, and people born in cities and large towns in Britain have an increased risk of death from

Table 8.8 Mean serum cholesterol concentrations according to abdominal circumference at birth in men and women aged 50–53 years

Abdominal circumference inches*	People (no.)	Total cholesterol (mmol/l)	Low density lipoprotein cholesterol (mmol/l)
≤ 11.5 (29.2)	53	6.7	4.5
− 12.0 (30.5)	43	6.9	4.6
− 12.5 (31.8)	31	6.8	4.4
− 13.0 (33.0)	45	6.2	4.0
> 13.0 (33.0)	45	6.1	4.0
Total	217	6.5	4.3

* Figures in parentheses are centimetres.
(This table was first published in the BMJ (Barker DJP, Martyn CN, Osmond C et al. Growth in utero and serum cholesterol concentrations in adult life. *British Medical Journal* 1993;**307**:1524-7) and is reproduced by permission of the BMJ)

chronic bronchitis irrespective of where they move to in later life, either within or outside the country.[51, 52] This suggests that the disease originates in part in early life. In Hertfordshire standardised mortality ratios for chronic bronchitis among men with birthweights of 2.5 kg or less were twice those among men with birthweights of more than 4.3 kg.

For many years there has been interest in the hypothesis that lower respiratory tract infection during infancy and early childhood predisposes to chronic airflow obstructions in later life.[53–57] The large geographical differences in death rates from chronic bronchitis in England and Wales are closely similar to the differences in infant deaths from respiratory infection earlier in this century.[58] Follow-up studies of individuals provide direct evidence that respiratory infection in early life has long-term effects. When the national sample of 3899 British children born in 1946 were studied as young adults those who had had one or more lower respiratory tract infections before 2 years of age had a higher prevalence of chronic cough.[59] A link between lower respiratory tract infection in early childhood and reduced lung function and death from chronic bronchitis in adult life has been shown in follow-up studies in Hertfordshire (Table 8.9) and Derbyshire.[60, 61]

This suggests that infancy may be a critical period in which infection may change lung function. Further evidence of the long-term effects of respiratory infection in early life came from a study of 70 year old men in Derbyshire, England, which also made use of health visitors' records.[61] The forced expiratory volume in 1 second (FEV_1) of men who had had pneumonia before the age of 2 years was 0.65 litres less than that of other men, a reduction in FEV_1 of approximately twice that associated with lifelong smoking.

Table 8.9   Mean forced expiratory volume in 1 second (FEV₁) litres, adjusted for height and age among men aged 59–67 years according to birthweight and the occurrence of bronchitis or pneumonia in infancy

Birthweight pounds*	Bronchitis or pneumonia in infancy†	
	Absent	Present
≤ 5.5 (2.5)	2.39 (22)	1.81 (4)
− 6.5 (2.9)	2.40 (70)	2.23 (10)
− 7.5 (3.4)	2.47 (163)	2.38 (25)
− 8.5 (3.9)	2.53 (179)	2.33 (12)
− 9.5 (4.3)	2.54 (103)	2.36 (5)
> 9.5 (4.3)	2.57 (43)	2.36 (3)
Total	2.50 (580)	2.30 (59)

* Figures in parentheses are kilograms.
† Figures in parentheses are numbers of men.
(This table was first published in the BMJ (Barker DJP, Godfrey KM, Fall C et al. Relation of birthweight and childhood respiratory infection to adult lung function and death from chronic obstructive airways disease. *British Medical Journal* 1991;**303**;671–5) and is reproduced by permission of the BMJ)

The simplest explanation of these observations is that infection of the lower respiratory tract during infancy has persisting deleterious effects which, added to the effects of poor airway growth *in utero*, predispose to the development of chronic bronchitis in later life. Factors implicated in "programming" of the respiratory system include fetal exposure to maternal smoking during pregnancy, and exposure to environmental allergens, or viral respiratory infections during infancy.[62] Although this paper has mainly focused on the role of nutrition in fetal health, it is clear that fetal health is influenced by many interrelated social factors.

Mothers and babies today: towards health improvement

The findings outlined here suggest that coronary heart disease (CHD), stroke, non-insulin dependent diabetes, hypertension, and chronic airflow obstruction originate *in utero*. Emerging evidence suggests that prenatal development may also contribute to other chronic diseases, such as osteoporosis,[63] cancers of the reproductive system,[64, 65] and schizophrenia.[66] Protecting the nutrition and health of young women and their babies must therefore be a priority. The history of Britain gives an insight into social conditions which have been harmful to mothers and babies in the past. Poverty, inadequate food, poor housing, and overcrowding led to the deaths of many infants, reduced the life expectancy of those who survived, and laid the foundations for today's inequalities in health.[67, 68]

Social conditions are improving, yet encouraged by the fashion industry, many young women today are unduly thin. The babies of thin women may be at increased risk of CHD, non-insulin dependent diabetes and raised blood pressure.[5, 15, 34–36, 69] Encouraged by sections of the food industry other young women today are unduly fat. The babies of women who are overweight may also be at increased risk of CHD and non-insulin dependent diabetes.[17, 70] The effects of a mother's body size are largely independent of its effects on the size of the baby. So too, it seems, are the effects of what she eats in pregnancy. Even famine has unexpectedly small effects on growth but the baby's physiology and metabolism are permanently altered.[71, 72]

Nutritional interventions in pregnancy

As yet, we do not know the true impact of maternal nutrition on fetal development. The relatively disappointing effects of nutritional interventions in pregnancy on birthweight in humans have led to the view that fetal development is little affected by changes in maternal nutrition. It is, however, clear that birthweight alone is an inadequate summary measure of fetal experience. We need a more sophisticated view of optimal fetal development which takes account of the long-term sequelae of fetal adaptations to undernutrition.

The Chief Medical Officer for Scotland has written:[73]

> At present we do not know whether it is more important to improve living conditions in adult life and try to persuade people to change their lifestyles, or to improve the health and nutrition of pregnant women and pre-school children. Obviously any sensible policy for improving (Scotland's) health must do both. But much depends on which is likely to yield greater long-term benefits, and at present we do not know. We are equally ignorant about the interactions that almost certainly exist between the enduring metabolic sequelae of inadequate nutrition early in life and unhealthy eating, drinking and exercise patterns in middle age.

Studies now in progress in Britain should help to resolve this. In Hertfordshire, the lifestyles of 5000 men and women, whose early growth was recorded, are now being documented. In Southampton 20,000 young women are being asked to take part in a study of diet and body composition. It is hoped that such studies will give some preliminary answers and inform the public health. For effective interventions to prevent or arrest disease we need, however, to progress beyond the epidemiological associations to greater understanding of the cellular and molecular processes that underlie them. We also need to know about how factors combine or interact over the life span, in order to help those who have had a poor start in early life avoid health consequences later in adulthood.

1 Barker DJP. Fetal origins of coronary heart disease. *British Medical Journal* 1995;**311**:171–4

2 Barker DJP, Osmond C. Infant mortality, childhood nutrition and ischaemic heart disease in England and Wales. *Lancet* 1986;**i**:1077–81

3 Local Government Board. *39th Annual Report 1909–10. Supplement on infant and child mortality.* 1910

4 McCance RA, Widdowson EM. The determinants of growth and form. *Proceedings of the Royal Society (Series B)* 1974;**185**:1–17

5 Barker DJP. *Mothers, Babies and Health in Later Life.* Edinburgh: Churchill Livingstone, 1998

6 Lucas A. Programming by early nutrition in man. In: Bock GR, Whelen J, eds. *The Childhood Environment and Adult Disease.* Chichester: Wiley, 1991

7 Fowden AL. Endocrine regulation of fetal growth. *Reproduction, Fertility and Development* 1995;**7**:351–63

8 Harding JE, Johnston BM. Nutrition and fetal growth. *Reproduction, Fertility and Development* 1995;**7**:539–47

9 Rudolph AM. The fetal circulation and its response to stress. *Journal of Developmental Physiology* 1984;**6**:11–19

10 Oliver MH, Harding JE, Breier BH, *et al.* Glucose but not a mixed amino acid infusion regulates plasma insulin-like growth factor-1 concentrations in fetal sheep. *Pediatric Research* 1993;**34**:62–5

11 Barker DJP, Osmond C, Simmonds SJ, *et al.* The relation of small head circumference and thinness at birth to death from cardiovascular disease in adult life. *British Medical Journal* 1993;**306**:422–6

12 Leon DA, Lithell H, Vagero D, *et al.* Biological and social influences on mortality in a cohort of 15,000 Swedes followed from birth to old age. *Journal of Epidemiology and Community Health* 1997;**51**:594

13 Frankel S, Elwood P, Sweetnam P, *et al.* Birthweight, body-mass index in middle age, and incident coronary heart disease. *Lancet* 1996;**348**:1478–80

14 Rich-Edwards JW, Stampfer MJ, Manson JE, *et al.* Birthweight and risk of cardiovascular disease in a cohort of women followed up since 1976. *British Medical Journal* 1997;**315**:396–400

15 Stein CE, Fall CHD, Kumaran K, *et al.* Fetal growth and coronary heart disease in South India. *Lancet* 1996;**348**:1269–73

16 Martyn CN, Barker DJP, Osmond C. Mothers' pelvic size, fetal growth, and death from stroke and coronary heart disease in men in the UK. *Lancet* 1996;**348**:1264–8

17 Forsen T, Eriksson JG, Tuomilehto J. Mother's weight in pregnancy and coronary heart disease in a cohort of Finnish men: follow-up study. *British Medical Journal* 1997;**315**:837–40

18 Karlberg J. A biologically-oriented mathematical model (ICP) for human growth. *Acta Paediatrica. Supplement* 1989;**350**:70–94

19 Kramer MS, Joseph KS. Commentary: enigma of fetal/infant origins hypothesis. *Lancet* 1996;**348**:1254–5

20 Paneth N, Susser M. Early origin of coronary heart disease (the "Barker hypothesis"). *British Medical Journal* 1995;**310**:411–12

21 Elford J, Whincup P, Shaper AG. Early life experience and adult cardiovascular disease: longitudinal and case-control studies. *International Journal of Epidemiology* 1991;**20**:833–44

22 Ben-Shlomo Y, Davey Smith G. Deprivation in infancy or in adult life: which is more important for mortality risk? *Lancet* 1991;**337**:530–4

23 Bartley M, Power C, Blane D, *et al.* Birthweight and later socio-economic disadvantage: evidence from the 1958 British Cohort Study. *British Medical Journal* 1994;**309**:1475–9

24 Law CM, Shiell AW. Is blood pressure inversely related to birthweight? The strength of evidence from a systematic review of the literature. *Journal of Hypertension* 1996;**14**:935–41

25 Hales CN, Barker DJP, Clark PMS, *et al.* Fetal and infant growth and impaired glucose tolerance at age 64. *British Medical Journal* 1991;**303**:1019–22

169

26 Koupilova I, Leon DA, Vagero D. Can confounding by socio-demographic and behavioural factors explain the association between size at birth and blood pressure at age 50 in Sweden? *Journal of Epidemiology and Community Health* 1997;**51**:14-18

27 Rose G. Sick individuals and sick populations. *International Journal of Epidemiology* 1985;**14**:32-8

28 Barker DJP, Godfrey KM, Osmond C, *et al.* The relation of fetal length, ponderal index and head circumference to blood pressure and the risk of hypertension in adult life. *Pediatric Perinatal Epidemiology* 1992;**6**:35-44

29 Barker DJP, Gluckman PD, Godfrey KM, *et al.* Fetal nutrition and cardiovascular disease in adult life. *Lancet* 1993;**341**:938-41

30 Langley SC, Jackson AA. Increased systolic blood pressure in adult rats induced by fetal exposure to maternal low protein diets. *Clinical Science* 1994;**86**:217-22

31 Petry CJ, Ozanne SE, Wang CL, *et al.* Early protein restriction and obesity independently induce hypertension in 1-year-old rats. *Clinical Science* 1997;**93**:147-52

32 Law CM, Barker DJP, Bull AR, *et al.* Maternal and fetal influences on blood pressure. *Archives of Disease in Childhood* 1991;**66**:1291-5

33 Whincup P, Cook D, Papacosta O, *et al.* Maternal factors and development of cardiovascular risk: evidence from a study of blood pressure in children. *Journal of Human Hypertension* 1994;**8**:337-43

34 Godfrey KM, Forrester T, Barker DJP, *et al.* The relation of maternal nutritional status during pregnancy to blood pressure in childhood. *British Journal of Obstetrics and Gynaecology* 1994;**101**:398-403

35 Clark PM, Atton C, Law CM, *et al.* Weight gain in pregnancy, triceps skinfold thickness and blood pressure in the offspring. *Obstetrics and Gynaecology* 1998;**91**:103-7

36 Margetts BM, Rowland MGM, Foord FA, *et al.* The relation of maternal weight to the blood pressures of Gambian children. *International Journal of Epidemiology* 1991;**20**:938-43

37 Campbell DM, Hall MH, Barker DJP, *et al.* Diet in pregnancy and the offspring's blood pressure 40 years later. *British Journal of Obstetrics and Gynaecology* 1996;**103**:273-80

38 Lever AF, Harrap SB. Essential hypertension: a disorder of growth with origins in childhood? *Journal of Hypertension* 1992;**10**:101-20

39 Fall CHD, Osmond C, Barker DJP, *et al.* Fetal and infant growth and cardiovascular risk factors in women. *British Medical Journal* 1995;**310**:428-32

40 Phipps K, Barker DJP, Hales CN, *et al.* Fetal growth and impaired glucose tolerance in men and women. *Diabetologia* 1993;**36**:225-8

41 Lithell HO, McKeigue PM, Berglund L, *et al.* Relation of size at birth to non-insulin dependent diabetes and insulin concentrations in men aged 50-60 years. *British Medical Journal* 1996;**312**:406-10

42 Olah KS. Low maternal birthweight - an association with impaired glucose tolerance in pregnancy. *Journal of Obstetrics and Gynaecology* 1996;**16**:5-8

43 Curhan GC, Willett WC, Rimm EB, *et al.* Birthweight and adult hypertension and diabetes mellitus in US men. *American Journal of Hypertension* 1996;**9**:11A(abstract)

44 McCance DR, Pettitt DJ, Hanson RL, *et al.* Birthweight and non-insulin dependent diabetes: thrifty genotype, thrifty phenotype, or surviving small baby genotype? *British Medical Journal* 1994;**308**:942-5

45 Law CM, Gordon GS, Shiell AW, *et al.* Thinness at birth and glucose tolerance in seven year old children. *Diabetic Medicine* 1995;**12**:24-9

46 Whincup PH, Cook DG, Adshead F, *et al.* Childhood size is more strongly related than size at birth to glucose and insulin levels in 10-11 year-old children. *Diabetologia* 1997;**40**:319-26

47 Taylor DJ, Thompson CH, Kemp GJ, *et al.* A relationship between impaired fetal growth and reduced muscle glycolysis revealed by ^{31}P magnetic resonance spectroscopy. *Diabetologia* 1995;**38**:1205-12

48 Bjorntorp P. Insulin resistance: the consequence of a neuroendocrine disturbance? *International Journal of Obesity* 1995;**19**(1 suppl):S6-S10

49 Barker DJP, Martyn CN, Osmond C, *et al.* Growth in utero and serum cholesterol concentrations in adult life. *British Medical Journal* 1993;**307**:1524-7

170

50 Martyn CN, Meade TW, Stirling Y, et al. Plasma concentrations of fibrinogen and factor VII in adult life and their relation to intra-uterine growth. *British Journal of Haematology* 1995;**89**:142-6

51 Reid DD, Fletcher CM. International studies in chronic respiratory disease. *British Medical Bulletin* 1971;**27**:59-64

52 Osmond C, Barker DJP, Slattery JM. Risk of death from cardiovascular disease and chronic bronchitis determined by place of birth in England and Wales. *Journal of Epidemiology and Community Health* 1990;**44**:139-41

53 Holland WW, Halil T, Bennett AE, et al. Factors influencing the onset of chronic respiratory disease. *British Medical Journal* 1969;**2**:205-8

54 Reid DD. The beginnings of bronchitis. *Proceedings of the Royal Society of Medicine* 1969;**62**:311-16

55 Samet JM, Tager IB, Speizer FE. The relationship between respiratory illness in childhood and chronic air-flow obstruction in adulthood. *American Review of Respiratory Diseases* 1983;**127**:508-23

56 Phelan PD. Does adult chronic obstructive lung disease really begin in childhood? *British Journal of Diseases of the Chest* 1984;**78**:1-9

57 Strachan DP. Do chesty children become chesty adults? *Archives of Disease in Childhood* 1990;**65**:161-2

58 Barker DJP, Osmond C. Childhood respiratory infection and adult chronic bronchitis in England and Wales. *British Medical Journal* 1987;**292**:1271-5

59 Mann SL, Wadsworth MEJ, Colley JRT. Accumulation of factors influencing respiratory illness in members of a national birth cohort and their offspring. *Journal of Epidemiology and Community Health* 1992;**46**:286-92

60 Barker DJP, Godfrey KM, Fall C, et al. Relation of birthweight and childhood respiratory infection to adult lung function and death from chronic obstructive airways disease. *British Medical Journal* 1991;**303**:671-5

61 Shaheen SO, Barker DJP, Shiell AW, et al. The relationship between pneumonia in early childhood and impaired lung function in late adult life. *American Journal of Respiratory and Critical Care Medicine* 1994;**149**:616-19

62 Dexateux C, Stocks J. Lung development and early origins of childhood respiratory illness. In: Marmont MG, Wadsworth MEJ, eds. Fetal and early childhood environment: long-term health implications. *British Medical Bulletin* 1997;**53**:740-57

63 Fall C, Hindmarsh P, Dennison E, et al. Programming of growth hormone secretion and bone mineral density in elderly men: an hypothesis. *Journal of Clinical Endocrinology and Metabolism* 1998;**83**:135-9

64 Barker DJP, Winter PD, Osmond C, et al. Weight gain in infancy and cancer of the ovary. *Lancet* 1995;**345**:1087-8

65 Michels KB, Trichopoulos D, Robins JM, et al. Birthweight as a risk factor for breast cancer. *Lancet* 1996;**348**:1542-6

66 Susser E, Neugebauer R, Hoeak W, et al. Schizophrenia after prenatal exposure to famine. *Lancet* 1999;(in press)

67 Barker DJP, Osmond C, Pannett B. Why Londoners have low death rates from ischaemic heart disease and stroke. *British Medical Journal* 1992;**305**:1551-4

68 Barker DJP, Osmond C. Inequalities in health in Britain: specific explanations in three Lancashire towns. *British Medical Journal* 1987;**294**:1351

69 Leger J, Levy-Marchal C, Bloch J, et al. Reduced final height and indications for insulin resistance in 20 year olds born small for gestational age: regional cohort study. *British Medical Journal* 1997;**315**:341-7

70 Fall CHD, Stein CE, Kumaran K, et al. Size at birth, maternal weight, and non-insulin dependent diabetes in South India. *Diabetic Medicine* 1998;**15**:220-7

71 Campbell DM, Hall MH, Barker DJP, et al. Diet in pregnancy and the offspring's blood pressure 40 years later. *British Journal of Obstetrics and Gynaecology* 1996;**103**:273-80

72 Ravelli ACJ, Van Der Meulen JHP, Michels RPJ, et al. Glucose tolerance in adults after prenatal exposure to famine. *Lancet* 1998;**351**:173-7

73 Kendall R. From the Chief Medical Officer. *Health Bulletin* 1993;**51**:351-2

171

ter 9 – Ensuring a healthy future for our children

The argument about our children's rights is based neither on institutional vested interests nor sentimentality about the young – it is based on the fact that childhood is a period when minds and bodies, values and personalities are being formed, and during which even temporary deprivation is capable of inflicting life-long damage and distortion on human development.

(JP Grant, 1994)

The evidence reviewed in this report has shown that child health is determined by a complex interaction of a large array of social, economic and personal factors. Child health is marred by inequalities and these inequities may be a result of the child's ethnic origin, their parents employment status, the type of housing and neighbourhood that they live in, or, most importantly, their social class background and the economic status of their family.[1] Kumar noted that since low income families tend to be multiply deprived, and often for long periods, the cumulative effect on their children's health is likely to be greater than that of any single indicator of deprivation.[2] Children who live in poverty will be at greater risk of poor health as infants, as young children, and for the rest of their lives.

The relationship between inequity and ill health is now well established but recent studies have revealed that inequity within the UK is increasing rather than decreasing,[3,4] The United Nations Development Programme considers that the UK is now one of the most unequal industrialised countries in the world.[5] The relationship between inequality and ill health is therefore more relevant than ever before.

There is a need to take a fresh look at the interventions and initiatives designed to reduce inequalities and to take account of the relationships that exist between social, economic, and health policy and to understand how they interact. Any successful intervention is likely to involve a combined

172

and pro-active package of social, economic and health policies which are centred on the child. This has policy implications at both the local and national level. National policies need to aim at reducing the income differentials in the UK which could be achieved via employment, education and economic policies and through the tax and benefits systems. Local policies need to consider housing provision, environment, public transport, and access to services. The needs of ethnic minority groups in relation to health and health inequalities require careful and sensitive consideration, including appropriate services to facilitate the treatment of those whose first language is not English. Because inequalities in health are the result of so many complex interactions, its solution must involve more than one agency. The health services alone cannot deal with the effects of poverty, and health interventions will only be effective if they are combined with socio-economic policies.

The need for interagency collaboration

At a local level, many services and sectors contribute to promoting young children's health. The four main services and sectors involved are primary health care, education services, social services, and the voluntary sector, but children's health will also be influenced by the adequacy of other local services, including council housing policy, provision for homeless families, parks, libraries, leisure services, etc.

Families often particularly appreciate the non-stigmatising help and advice about their children which they may be offered in ordinary community settings such as a nursery or baby clinic. Most families will need such advice about their children at some stage, but some, facing multiple adversities, need longer-term, multiservice interventions to minimise the risk of their children developing established emotional and behavioural problems. It is these families who benefit most from integrated interagency planning across all the children's services, including education, social services, primary and other health care, and the voluntary sector. Where professionals or voluntary workers in an area are aware of a range of resources, developed as part of a comprehensive review, families are more likely to find appropriate and accessible help.

Barriers to interagency collaboration

The emphasis on interagency collaboration has been an increasingly prominent theme of legislation over the last 10 years. The Children Act (1989)[6] and subsequent guidance required local authorities to review day care and childminding provision for children in need every 3 years. This review was intended to involve health authorities, voluntary organisations,

173

the private sector, employers, and parents. In 1996 further legislation required local authorities to produce 3-yearly Children's Services Plans[7] in conjunction and partnership with education services, the voluntary sector and health services. Several of the new government initiatives, such as Sure Start, the Child Care strategy and the Action Zones have interagency and private public partnership as essential aspects of their organisation.

However, in practice it has proved difficult to break down barriers between different agencies. Malek[8] has identified some of the obstacles which have interfered with interprofessional collaboration in health services.

For example, the various agencies and sectors:

• have different perceptions and terminologies concerning health;
• have different values and priorities, and a lack of shared objectives;
• have little experience of undertaking collaborative work at any stage – commissioning, planning, purchasing or providing;
• operate within different legislative frameworks, and the demands of legislative change have contributed to agencies becoming preoccupied in their particular field at the expense of joint work;
• have a lack of knowledge and understanding about other services and their contribution to child and adolescent health.

Breaking down the barriers to effective interagency collaboration

There are a number of developments which, if implemented, could accelerate the breakdown of barriers to interagency collaboration.

First, further common funding arrangements could be introduced. The Sure Start programme is innovative in that it is administered at government level, by a single budget managed by a committee drawn from different government departments. Early years services across the various sectors, including those relating to children's health, could also be managed from a single budget. This would necessitate clear prioritisation and jointly determined strategic planning.

Second, in order to break down barriers between professional groups, and increase understanding and awareness of each other's professional roles, more multidisciplinary training both undergraduate and post-graduate should be introduced. For example, in the field of mental health, short and longer courses in behavioural, counselling and family therapy techniques are available, a diploma in promoting young children's mental health has been developed,[9] and a masters degree in infant mental health is now available from the Tavistock Clinic in North London.

The importance of accessible and acceptable services

However carefully planned, services with a role in promoting young children's health, or in preventing emotional and behavioural problems, will only be effective where parents want them and use them. The importance of careful needs assessment, in partnership with parents, cannot be underestimated. Organisations should be carefully monitored to ensure that they are offering services which are actually reaching those parents and children in need. The following evaluative checklist has been proposed.[10]

In relation to their target group, effective services should be:

- available;
- acceptable;
- accessible;
- affordable;
- accountable;
- appropriate;
- across-agency.

This list emphasises the importance of providing services which do not exclude families because of cultural, religious or language differences.

One approach to minimising such exclusion is to involve linkworkers from the target community, who can help families access mainstream services. Providing linkworkers for pregnant Pakistani women who had had a previous low birthweight baby has been shown to be associated with several positive outcomes, including increased birthweight and fewer feeding problems relative to a control group.[11] Where professionals and families are using different conceptual frameworks to explain, for example, the causes of and appropriate treatment for children's emotional and behavioural problems, linkworkers do not simply translate language but can also facilitate intercultural understanding.

Another way of providing services for groups who may be excluded from mainstream service delivery, involves the development of specific projects with the needs of particular groups in mind. An example is shown in the box overleaf.

Evaluating effectiveness

Demonstrating that parents like a service is of course only one consideration for service planners – of equal importance is evidence that a particular intervention actually has, or is likely to have, a beneficial impact on young children's health. Ensuring that projects are developed with outcome indicators integral to the design is particularly important in the face of so many new initiatives. In terms of measuring health outcomes for young children, there is a tension between delivering specific interventions to certain parents, where effectiveness can be measured using randomised controlled trials, and multifaceted interventions which aim to alter the ecology of a community so that levels of health problems and inequalities are reduced. An example follows below.

175

The Moyenda Project

This project was established in London in 1991 by the charity Exploring Parenthood, with 3-year funding from the Department of Health and various charitable trusts. It had three main aims. First, it aimed to organise parent support groups within both the Asian community and also the African-Carribean community, involving parents, and existing black community groups as much as possible in the session planning. Second, it developed a questionnaire survey of both black parents' needs for support services and family support professionals' perceptions of their black clients' needs. Third, it aimed to produce relevant support materials which could be used by parents and family support professionals to address the concerns of black parents. Particularly in the work with Asian families, the most effective way to offer parenting groups was found to involve training local community volunteers as group facilitators. The project was well received by both parents and communities, with a high demand for further culturally sensitive support groups to be provided. The Moyenda Project is now in the process of evolving into an independent black-led organisation involving a network of black professionals providing a variety of parenting and family initiatives.[12]

The strategic aims of both child health services and the personal social services with respect to the welfare of children are broadly similar. Local authorities are responsible for ensuring that children in need are provided with the help they require in order that they attain a reasonable standard of health and development.[13] Child health services seek to ensure that as many children as possible reach adulthood with their potential as uncompromised as possible by illness, environmental hazard or unhealthy lifestyle.[14] The welfare of children depends on both health and social services utilising strategies of proven effectiveness, within a context of well co-ordinated structures, to achieve these joint aims. Voluntary child care agencies are well placed to assist these aims in association with both these sectors, by close involvement in the joint planning process and by challenging professional boundaries that impede the promotion of children's welfare.

We do not believe that children's welfare can best be served by major changes that focus on redistributing duties between the health and social services. We believe that rather than seeking solutions through large scale organisational change, the welfare of children can be best promoted through jointly agreed clear and measurable outcomes and defining the role of respective agencies, including the voluntary and private sectors, in pursuing these outcomes.

Factors that impede children's development are strongly interconnected. Poorly looked after children suffer from disproportionately high health related problems. Poverty and low standards of parental education are associated with low birthweight and subsequently higher levels of psychoso-

Better Beginnings, Better Futures Project

This Canadian government funded project is an example of targeted service development where evaluation of effectiveness is integral to the project. As such it serves as a potential model for the Sure Start programme. The Better Beginnings, Better Futures project aims to demonstrate the effectiveness of a set of strategic interventions designed to prevent serious social, emotional, behavioural, physical and cognitive problems in young children, while promoting their social, emotional, behavioural, physical and cognitive development. The interventions are focused specifically on socio-economically disadvantaged communities. The project is targeted at children aged 0–4 in eight communities, with a further three similar communities targeting 4–8 year old children. Five of these communities are First Nation communities. Government funding is used to provide additional services in each of the project areas. The exact combination of services in each area is determined through liaison between local steering committees, government representatives and project researchers, and is selected to meet local needs from a menu of potential service developments. Home visiting is part of all projects targeting 0–4 year olds, and classroom enrichment is part of all projects for 4–8 year olds. Child care enrichment is provided in all participating communities. Child development programmes, parent training and support, community development, and community healing (an established tradition in First Nation Communities) are optional components of the programmes. The projects are designed to compare 4 year olds in the chosen communities when the projects began with 4 year olds who have completed the 0–4 programme, and to do the same with 8 year olds, using parent and teacher report and direct testing. Community indicators, for example, rates of child protection, will also be assessed. Some children will be followed for 20 years to ascertain long-term outcomes. Children from matched communities where the programme does not run will also be followed for the duration of the programme, and some for 20 years. The cost of each component of the programme will be monitored to allow for cost/benefit analyses to be made.[15]

cial problems. Poor school attendance and performance can be expected to result in earlier pregnancies, increased levels of delinquency, and worse adult health. Failure of any individual agency to discharge its duties effectively will inevitably impact upon other sectors.

An improvement in co-ordination between child welfare services to maximise their "value" to children and families was the main strategic recommendation of the Audit Commission report, *Seen But Not Heard*.[16] While progress has been inevitably patchy, local authorities have made considerable strides in improving both the formulation of joint aims and co-ordination of services through the medium of Children's Services Plans (CSPs). We believe that the continuing development of CSPs, especially through the adoption of specific jointly agreed outcome measures, will increase the accountability, visibility and clarity of agency operations. CSPs should be the main medium through which the goals of statutory agencies with respect to children's welfare should be expressed. The strategic activities of individual agencies must be geared to the aims expressed in CSPs.

Effective planning cannot take place without careful consideration of the views of both parents and children. Users of services are sources of essential information. Failure to develop methods to consult users and give equal weight to their views will fatally compromise the integrity of the most well co-ordinated strategy.

Joint strategic planning depends on information systems that deliver a volume and specificity of information appropriate to the decision making process. Better exchange of information between as well as within, agencies is essential to ensure that progress towards joint targets is maintained. More emphasis is also needed on the use of management information in the prospective reallocation of resources and not just for the purpose of monitoring compliance to procedures.

Joint planning will not in itself lead to better outcomes for children. More emphasis needs to be given to the adoption of effective procedures and, by implication, the abandonment of ineffective ones. Collaborating agencies need a common understanding of evidence based practice and the need to both commission and deliver interventions that are based on the best possible evidence that the chosen intervention is likely to result in an outcome that promotes children's health and welfare.

Speaking at the 1998 Annual Edward Chadwick lecture, Richard Smith, Editor of the *British Medical Journal*, revealed the findings of an expert group who assessed a range of studies on health inequalities and ranked the measures they recommended according to their chances of success. The group recommended 10 interventions that are most likely to help reduce health inequalities between the rich and poor, after assessing a range of options covering areas such as mother and child health, housing, nutrition, education, and mental health. A complex formula was used to assess the strength of the evidence, the scale of the likely benefit, the fit with government policy, and the ease and cost of implementation. The group's recommendations concentrate on relatively small interventions, rather than macro-changes, and included a number of child-centred recommendations including preschool education and child care, support for new mothers around childbirth to promote breastfeeding and mental health, accident prevention, and free school milk (Smith R, Edward Chadwick Lecture, Manchester, October 1998, personal communication).

All government policies and programmes, whether directly concerned with children or not, should be evaluated as far as possible for their impact on children.[1] Many other government policies, such as transport, housing, environment, employment, and fiscal/welfare policies, will have effects on children. Unfortunately, however, these effects are often overlooked. Social

178

policy especially will have a major impact on child health. Government policy needs to recognise the difficulties parents, especially lone parents, have in balancing earning with caring and should be equally supportive of those who choose to spend an extended period at home (requiring provision of adequately paid parental leave) and those who choose to return to work.

Mitigating the effects of inequalities in health

Following the recommendation of the 1976 Court report *Fit for the Future*,[17] the Children's Committee was set up in 1978 for a period of 3 years under the chairmanship of Professor Brimblecombe. The remit included the "co-ordination and development of health and social services as they relate to children and families with children". It was the only government advisory body which examined all aspects of policy and legislation for their impact on children in an interdisciplinary way. The committee felt that a broad kind of advocacy of children's interests was needed if any impact was to be made on public and parliamentary opinion. In those 3 years, a number of papers were produced, including reports on perinatal mortality, the under fives, and corporal punishment. In all of these activities, the importance of working across the boundaries that existed between services, departments and communities was established. The Committee's demise left a serious gap which was reflected when the white paper *The Health of the Nation*[10] was published in 1992, and none of the key issues included a specific mention of children. In the new environment made possible by the government's latest 1998 green paper *Our Healthier Nation*,[19] there is another opportunity for consideration of an independent voice for all children. Two Nordic countries, Sweden and Norway, have a Children Ombudsman. These concepts could be extended to the UK to an independent Children's Commissioner, whose role would be to promote the rights and interests of children and young people. Much current policy making and practice in the UK in areas which affect children do not give enough recognition to their rights and interests. Introducing a Commissioner would also help the UK government to fulfil its obligations under the UN Convention on the Rights of the Child that children's rights receive political priority.[20]

The UK has started to move towards this way of tackling the challenges of inequity. The government publication *The Health of the Nation*[18] focused more on individual health related behaviours (such as smoking, diet, etc.) and there was a lack of consideration of national macro-economic policies and policies for children. By contrast, the follow-up report *Our Healthier Nation* has placed a much greater emphasis on social inequality and its contribution to disease.[19] Health inequality research projects totalling £1.7

million have recently been commissioned by the Department of Health. These include increasing breastfeeding among low uptake groups to reduce social, ethnic, and regional variations in health; a randomised controlled trial looking at the effect of out-of-home day care on the health and welfare of socially disadvantaged families with children and a systematic review into inequalities in mental health.[21]

The government has also accepted the principles in the Health Committee's reports that the health needs of children are significantly different from those of adults and effective health services for children will depend on these needs being understood. Health services need to be specifically tailored to children's needs.[22] The government has also launched a £540 million Sure Start programme which aims to tackle social exclusion for the most vulnerable young children and their families. This initiative demonstrates the government's recognition of the need for social support for parents within their communities requiring provision of a range of high quality, affordable child care options. The children of lone parents are at greater risk of a range of health problems associated with poverty. The main focus of the programme will be investing in preventing social exclusion. It will work with parents to ensure that their children are healthy, confident and ready to learn when they reach school. Help will begin with a visit from an outreach worker within 3 months of the baby's birth. This will allow an assessment of the needs of the child and provide advice and support for the parents. A range of services will be available, including advice on breastfeeding and support for children with learning difficulties and emotional and behavioural difficulties,[23] although we would not expect this to replace the invaluable work of health visitors. Investment in early childhood promises high value in reducing health inequalities and promoting educational achievement and attainment. Spencer found that countries, both developed and less developed, which had pursued social policies aimed at reducing income disparity and supporting the poor and vulnerable have succeeded in reducing poverty and its health conse-quences.[24] The long-term benefit of such policies are likely to far outweigh the short-term costs.

Although we have highlighted in this report specific areas where there is a relationship between inequality and health, the relationship is a complex one and there will be a range of interlinking factors preventing individuals from achieving better health and well-being. A multifaceted approach is therefore needed, as tackling particular factors in isolation will not achieve the desired outcome of reversing the trend in the UK towards an increasingly inequitable society.

Health and welfare services should be concerted in their commitment to the health of children through clear evidenced and responsible programmes of education and care that particularly target social, ethnic or illness groups that may be at risk. It is important that the improvements and interventions mentioned in this report are implemented and are not regarded as justification for further study. The necessity for this focused yet holistic approach involves health care.

Recommendations

National Policy

1. We support and adopt the World Medical Association Declaration of Ottawa on the Right of the Child to Healthcare. All organisations, professions and institutions should ensure that any work done with, or on behalf, of children, or affecting children's well-being, conforms to this Declaration and that of the United Nations Convention on the Rights of the Child.
2. We recommend the introduction of an independent Children's Commissioner, with separate but linked commissioners for England, Northern Ireland, Scotland and Wales. The role of the commissioner would be to ensure that any new government policies which may have an effect on children are evaluated with respect to their impact on children's rights, interests, and health.
3. We recommend that steps are taken to maintain and extend the government's commitment to tackle social exclusion through education and fiscal measures.
4. All families should continue to be entitled to child benefit payments and we recommend that the government should not consider any further cuts to lone parent benefit, which will disproportionately affect children in greatest need.
5. We recommend that the government's Welfare to Work policy recognises the particular problems of lone parents in the workforce, and that further encouragement, including fiscal incentives, are given to employers who adopt family friendly policies (that is, creches, flexitime, opportunities to work from home, etc.). The government should consider introducing increased entitlement to maternity leave and the introduction of a right to paternity leave for all parents.
6. A good general education appears to help young women avoid early motherhood, taking up smoking, and smoking during pregnancy. We commend current efforts in prioritising education, and recommend that further steps are taken to improve educational opportunities and outcomes for children from low income families.
7. The BMA welcomes the recent White Paper on tobacco control but continues to recommend that the government take firm regulatory action in implementing a complete ban on tobacco advertising and smoking in public places.

181

8. More effective interventions are required to discourage alcohol consumption and the use of illicit drugs by parents or carers which poses a health risk to children in their care.

9. The BMA welcomes the government's decision to review the law on the physical punishment of children by parents and their carers. We believe that physical punishment is inefficient, ineffective and harmful in modifying children's behaviour and that parents should be encouraged and assisted in developing other methods of child discipline.

10. We recommend that the professional registration of health visitors should be safeguarded to enable them to continue to deliver a comprehensive and skilled service to children and families.

11. Children should be seen as important contributors to our understandings of appropriate care and their views should be taken into consideration when developing NHS services.

Health policy and interventions

12. We welcome recent government initiatives such as Sure Start and the National Family and Parenting Institute and recommend that they are supported, with effective training and supervision for those involved in delivering services to families, and with continued monitoring and evaluation of child outcomes.

13. A national agenda to reduce the risk of child injury is required. Enforcement of existing legislation on speed limits, seatbelt usage, and infant car restraints are as important as new initiatives.

14. Efforts need to be maintained to emphasise parents' responsibility for postnatal protection of their children from passive smoking, and to encourage them to quit smoking, for example, offering smokers who wish to quit free nicotine replacement therapy where appropriate.

15. We recommend that children should be encouraged to be physically active from an early age. However, road traffic presents a major risk for children's health and safety and all relevant government departments should facilitate and promote active play in a safe environment, establish traffic free zones, safe walk to school routes, cycling lanes, and play streets.

16. We recommend that immunisation services for children against childhood diseases should be promoted and maintained according to the current advice from the Joint Committee on Vaccination and Immunisation. Government should work in a co-operative manner with doctors to encourage participation.

17. We recommend that all water companies should be legally obliged to ensure adequate fluoride levels in their water supplies. (Optimum level of one part of fluoride per million parts of water 1 ppm.)

18. We recommend that separate and suitably equipped facilities for the reception and treatment of children should be available in all accident and emergency departments. Doctors and nurses in this setting should receive training about basic child development; at the very least there should be a paediatric liaison doctor and nurse available.

19. We recommend that the uptake of antenatal testing for HIV be increased so that women have the opportunity to benefit from interventions such as antiretroviral therapy, caesarean section and breastfeeding advice, thereby significantly reducing the risk of their children being infected.

Nutrition

20. We recommend that ensuring good standards of nutrition and advice on healthy eating for young women and their babies must be a priority for government action with the provision of a safety net for children at nutritional risk, for example, by providing free nursery and school milk, fruit, and a balanced main meal.

21. We recommend the development of a government led strategy to improve the diets of infants and young children and help prevent anaemia, dental caries, and obesity. Particular efforts should be focused on increasing breastfeeding rates and improving the quality of weaning diets; breastfeeding should be actively promoted by government and health professionals, to employers as well as to parents, and the benefits monitored.

22. The school curriculum should include nutrition and cooking skills with a special emphasis on providing healthy meals on a low income.

Local policy

23. All children with disabilities should have the right to be included in their local community, attend local facilities including leisure facilities, and mainstream school; these facilities must be well funded and resourced to meet their special needs.

24. We recommend equity in service provision, so that children with learning disabilities can expect equal access to the same treatment as other children.

25. Health authorities should initiate health visitor led identification of postnatal depression and specific training should be offered.

26. Health authorities and local authorities should collectively review their existing day care provision and develop, where necessary, collaborative programmes that act as a "one-stop-shop" for children and their families to gain access to health, education, and social services.

Inter-agency collaboration

27. We recommend that Child and Adolescent Mental Health Services (CAMHS) should become more involved in offering training and consultation to other health professionals and other agency workers in contact with children. All child health services should have strong child mental health professional support and mental health professionals should be attached to family practices and work with health visitors.
28. We recommend that the number of moves for children in public care should be kept to an absolute minimum, and that they are given a level of care and opportunities to compensate for their poor start in life.
29. The BMA supports the work of the voluntary child care agencies who are well placed to assist in encouraging interagency collaboration, by close involvement in the joint planning process and by dissolving professional boundaries that impede promotion of children's welfare.

Research

30. Research is required to identify what constitutes good quality child care for 0–5 year olds either within or outside of the home. In order to ensure maximum benefit from new initiatives, this must include robust evaluation of provision of their relative costs.
31. Research is needed that evaluates a wide range of child outcomes where income supplements have been offered to low income families.
32. Better evidence and dissemination of "what works" for children with emotional and behavioural problems, including the identification of the most effective interventions, and the age(s) at which these might be fruitful is required.
33. Further research into the full impact of maternal nutrition on fetal development is needed, which takes account of the long-term effects of fetal adaptations to undernutrition.
34. Research is required to understand the causes and long-term consequences of fatness in childhood, and to understand what influences from childhood affect obesity in later life.
35. Further studies are required to identify effective interventions that establish "what works" in supporting parents to quit smoking in pregnancy and beyond.
36. Further research is required to elucidate why such large numbers of children today need help for speech and language difficulties.
37. Further research into the increased incidence of asthma is required.

Future information needs

38. We recommend that an annual report on the health of children, similar to the Chief Medical Officer's report *On the State of the Public Health*,

should be published by the Department of Health with a view to monitoring health trends in children so that remedial action can be taken where needed and progress monitored.

1 Holtermann S. *All Our Futures: the impact of public expenditure and fiscal policies on Britain's children and young people.* Essex: Barnardos,1995

2 Kumar V. *Poverty and Inequality in the UK: the effects on children.* London: National Children's Bureau, 1996

3 Office for National Statistics. *Social Trends 27.* London: The Stationery Office, 1997

4 Department of Health. *Independent Inquiry into Inequalities in Health Report.* London: The Stationery Office, 1998

5 United Nations Development Programme. *Human Development Report 1996.* New York: Oxford University Press, 1996

6 House of Commons. *The Children Act 1989.* London: HMSO, 1989

7 Department of Health and Department for Education and Employment. *Children's Services Planning Guidance.* London: DH/DFEE, 1996

8 Malek M. *Nurturing Healthy Minds: the importance of the voluntary sector in promoting young people's mental health.* London: National Children's Bureau, 1997

9 Earle J, Hill P. *Theory into Practice: promoting the mental health of young children. Distance learning pack for health visitors.* London: St George's Hospital Medical School, 1998

10 Sinclair R, Hearn B, Pugh G. *Preventive Work with Families: the role of mainstream services.* London: National Children's Bureau, 1997

11 Dance J. A social intervention by linkworkers to Pakistani women, and pregnancy outcome (unpublished, 1987). Described in: Oakley A. *Social Support and Motherhood.* Oxford: Blackwell, 1992

12 Moyenda Project. *Exploring Parenthood.* London, 1995

13 House of Commons. *Children Act 1989.* London: HMSO, 1989

14 Department of Health. *Child Health in the Community: a guide to good practice.* London: Department of Health, 1995

15 Peters R, Crill Russell C. Promoting development and preventing disorder. The Better Beginnings, Better Futures Project. In: Peters R, McMahon R, eds. *Preventing Childhood Disorders, Substance Abuse and Delinquency.* London: Sage, 1996

16 Audit Commission. *Seen But Not Heard: co-ordinating community child health and social services for children in need.* London: HMSO, 1994

17 Secretary of State for Social Services, Secretary of State for Education and Science, Secretary of State for Wales. *Fit for the Future. Report of the Committee of Child Health Services,* vols 1, 2. London: HMSO, 1976

18 Department of Health. *The Health of the Nation.* London: HMSO, 1992

19 Department of Health. *Our Healthier Nation: Green Paper.* CM3852. London: The Stationery Office, 1998

20 Rosenbaum M, Newell P. *Taking Children Seriously. A proposal for a Children's Rights Commissioner.* London: Calouste Gulbenkian Foundation, 1991

21 Department of Health. Inequalities in Health. Press Release 6/5/98

22 Department of Health. *Government Response to the Reports of the Health Committee on Health Services for Children and Young People. Session 1996–1997.* London: Department of Health, 1997

23 Department for Education and Employment. Investing in Our Children. Press Release, 23 July 1998

24 Spencer N. *Poverty and Child Health.* Oxford: Radcliffe Medical Press, 1996

APPENDIX I

The United Nations Convention on the Rights of the Child

Abstract taken from The United Nations Convention on the Rights of the Child. Adopted by the General Assembly of the United Nations on 20 November 1989

Article 22

1. States Parties shall take appropriate measures to ensure that a child who is seeking refugee status or who is considered a refugee in accordance with applicable international or domestic law and procedures shall, whether unaccompanied or accompanied by his or her parents or by any other person, receive appropriate protection and humanitarian assistance in the enjoyment of applicable rights set forth in the present Convention and in other international human rights or humanitarian instruments to which the said States are Parties.
2. For this purpose, States Parties shall provide, as they consider appropriate, co-operation in any efforts by the United Nations and other competent intergovernmental organizations or non-governmental organizations co-operating with the United Nations to protect and assist such a child and to trace the parents or other members of the family of any refugee child in order to obtain information necessary for reunification with his or her family. In cases where no parents or other members of the family can be found, the child shall be accorded the same protection as any other child permanently or temporarily deprived of his or her family environment for any reason, as set forth in the present Convention.

Article 23

1. States Parties recognize that a mentally or physically disabled child should enjoy a full and decent life, in conditions which ensure dignity, promote self-reliance, and facilitate the child's active participation in the community.
2. States Parties recognize the right of the disabled child to special care and shall encourage and ensure the extension, subject to available resources, to the eligible child and those responsible for his or her care, of

assistance for which application is made and which is appropriate to the child's condition and to the circumstances of the parents or others caring for the child.

3. Recognizing the special needs of a disabled child, assistance extended in accordance with paragraph two of the present article shall be provided free of charge, whenever possible, taking into account the financial resources of the parents or others caring for the child, and shall be designed to ensure that the disabled child has effective access to and receives education, training, health care services, rehabilitation services, preparation for employment and recreation opportunities in a manner conducive to the child's achieving the fullest possible social integration and individual development, including his or her cultural and spiritual development.

4. States Parties shall promote, in the spirit of international co-operation, the exchange of appropriate information in the field of preventive health care and of medical, psychological and functional treatment of disabled children, including dissemination of and access to information concerning methods of rehabilitation, education and vocational services, with the aim of enabling States Parties to improve their capabilities and skills and to widen their experience in these areas. In this regard, particular account shall be taken of the needs of developing countries.

Article 24

1. States Parties recognize the right of the child to the enjoyment of the highest attainable standard of health and to facilities for the treatment of illness and rehabilitation of health. States Parties shall strive to ensure that no child is deprived of his or her right of access to such health care services.

2. States Parties shall pursue full implementation of this right and, in particular, shall take appropriate measures:
   (a) To diminish infant and child mortality;
   (b) To ensure the provision of necessary medical assistance and health care to all children with emphasis on the development of primary health care;
   (c) To combat disease and malnutrition including within the framework of primary health care, through *inter alia* the application of readily available technology and through the provision of adequate nutritious foods and clean drinking water, taking into consideration the dangers and risks of environmental pollution;
   (d) To ensure appropriate prenatal and postnatal health care for mothers;
   (e) To ensure that all segments of society, in particular parents and children, are informed, have access to education and are supported

in the use of basic knowledge of child health and nutrition, the advantages of breastfeeding, hygiene and environmental sanitation and the prevention of accidents;

(f) To develop preventive health care, guidance for parents and family planning education and services.

3. States Parties shall take all effective and appropriate measures with a view to abolishing traditional practices prejudicial to the health of children.

4. States Parties undertake to promote and encourage international co-operation with a view to achieving progressively the full realization of the right recognized in the present article. In this regard, particular account shall be taken of the needs of developing countries.

Article 25

States Parties recognize the right of a child who has been placed by the competent authorities for the purposes of care, protection or treatment of his or her physical or mental health, to a periodic review of the treatment provided to the child and all other circumstances relevant to his or her placement.

Article 26

1. States Parties shall recognize for every child the right to benefit from social security, including social insurance, and shall take the necessary measures to achieve the full realization of this right in accordance with their national law.

2. The benefits should, where appropriate, be granted, taking into account the resources and the circumstances of the child and persons having responsibility for the maintenance of the child, as well as any other consideration relevant to an application for benefits made by or on behalf of the child.

Article 27

1. States Parties recognize the right of every child to a standard of living adequate for the child's physical, mental, spiritual, moral and social development.

2. The parent(s) or others responsible for the child have the primary responsibility to secure, within their abilities and financial capacities, the conditions of living necessary for the child's development.

3. States Parties, in accordance with national conditions and within their means, shall take appropriate measures to assist parents and others

responsible for the child to implement this right and shall in case of need provide material assistance and support programmes, particularly with regard to nutrition, clothing and housing.

4. States Parties shall take all appropriate measures to secure the recovery of maintenance for the child from the parents or other persons having financial responsibility for the child, both within the State Party and from abroad. In particular, where the person having financial responsibility for the child lives in a State different from that of the child, States Parties shall promote the accession to international agreements or the conclusion of such agreements, as well as the making of other appropriate arrangements.

APPENDIX II

World Medical Association Declaration on the Right of the Child to Health Care

Preamble

1. The health care of a child, whether at home or in hospital, includes medical, emotional, social and financial aspects which interact in the healing process and which require special attention to the rights of the child as a patient.
2. Article 24 of the 1989 United Nations Convention on the Rights of the Child recognises the right of the child to the enjoyment of the highest attainable standard of health and to facilities for the treatment of illness and rehabilitation of health, and states that nations shall strive to ensure that no child is deprived of his or her right of access to such health care services.
3. In the context of this Declaration a child signifies a human being between the time of birth and the end of her/his seventeenth year, unless under the law applicable in the country concerned children reach their majority at some other age.

General Principles

4. Every child has an inherent right to life, as well as the right of access to the appropriate facilities for health promotion, the prevention and treatment of illness and the rehabilitation of health. Physicians and other health care providers have a responsibility to acknowledge and promote these rights, and to urge the material and human resources to uphold and fulfil them. In particular every effort should be made:

    (i) to protect to the maximum extent possible the survival and development of the child, and to recognise that parents (or legally entitled representatives) have primary responsibility for the development of the child and that both parents have common responsibilities in this respect;

    (ii) to ensure that the best interests of the child shall be the primary consideration in health care;

    (iii) to resist any discrimination in the provision of medical assistance and health care from considerations of age, gender, disease or disability, creed, ethnic origin, nationality, political affiliation, race, sexual orientation, or the social standing of the child or her/his parents or legally entitled representatives;

(iv) to attain suitable pre- and post-natal health care for the mother and child;

(v) to secure for every child the provision of adequate medical assistance and health care, including appropriate procedures to avoid pain, with emphasis on primary health care, on pertinent psychiatric care for those children with such needs and on care relevant to the special needs of disabled children;

(vi) to protect every child from unnecessary diagnostic procedures, treatment and research;

(vii) to combat disease and malnutrition;

(viii) to develop preventive health care;

(ix) to eradicate child abuse in its various forms; and

(x) to eradicate traditional practices prejudicial to the health of the child.

Specific Principles

Quality of care

5. Continuity and quality of care should be ensured by the team providing health care for a child.

6. Physicians and others providing health care to children should have the special training and skills necessary to enable them to respond appropriately to the medical, physical, emotional and developmental needs of children and their families.

7. In circumstances where a choice must be made between potential child patients for particular treatment which is in limited supply, the individual patients should be guaranteed a fair selection procedure for that treatment made on medical criteria alone and without discrimination.

Freedom of choice

8. The parents or legally entitled representatives, or where the child is of sufficient maturity the child herself/himself, should be able: to choose freely and to change the child's physician; to be satisfied that the physician of choice is free to make clinical and ethical judgements without any outside interference; and to ask for a second opinion of another physician at any stage.

Consent and self-determination

9. A child patient and her/his parents or legally entitled representatives have a right to active informed participation in all decisions involving the child's health care. The wishes of the child should be taken into account in such decision making, and should be given increasing weight dependent on her/his capacity of understanding. The mature child, in the judgement of the physician, is entitled to make her/his own decisions about health care.

10. Except in an emergency (see paragraph 12), informed consent is necessary before beginning any diagnostic process or therapy on a child, especially where it is an invasive procedure. In the majority of cases the consent shall be obtained from the parents or legally entitled representatives, although any wishes expressed by the child should be taken into account before consent is given. However, if the child is of sufficient maturity and understanding, the informed consent shall be obtained from the child herself/himself.

11. In general, a competent child patient and her/his parents or legally entitled representatives are entitled to withhold consent to any procedure or therapy. While it is presumed that parents or legally entitled representatives will act in the best interests of the child, occasionally this may not be so. Where a parent or legally entitled representative refuses consent to a procedure on, and/or treatment of, a child without which the child's health would be put in grave and irreversible danger and to which there is no alternative within the spectrum of generally accepted medical care the physician should obtain the relevant judicial or other legal authorization to perform such a procedure or treatment.

12. If the child is unconscious, or otherwise incapable of giving consent, and a parent or legally entitled representative is not available, but a medical intervention is needed urgently, then specific consent to the intervention may be presumed, unless it is obvious and beyond any reasonable doubt on the basis of a previous firm expression or conviction that consent to intervention would be refused in the particular situation (subject to the proviso detailed in paragraph 7).

13. A child patient and her/his parents or legally entitled representatives are entitled to refuse to participate in research or in the teaching of medicine. Such refusal must never interfere with the patient–physician relationship or jeopardize the child's medical care or other benefits to which she/he is entitled.

Access to information

14. The child patient and (except in the circumstances outlined in paragraph 18) her/his parents or legally entitled representatives are

entitled to be fully informed about her/his health status and medical condition, provided this would not be contrary to the interests of the child. However, confidential information in the child's medical record about a third party should not be provided to the child, the parents or the legally entitled representatives without the consent of that third party.

15. Any information should be provided in a manner appropriate to the culture and to the level of understanding of the recipient. This is particularly important in the case of information provided to the child, who should have the right of access to general health information.

16. Exceptionally, certain information may be withheld from the child, or her/his parents or legally entitled representatives, when there is good reason to believe that this information would create a serious hazard to the life or health of the child or to the physical or mental health of a person other than the child.

Confidentiality

17. In general the obligation of physicians and other health care workers to maintain the confidentiality of identifiable personal and medical information of patients (including information about health status, medical condition, diagnosis, prognosis, and treatment) applies as much in the case of child patients as it does for those who are adult.

18. The child patient mature enough to be unaccompanied at a consultation by her/his parents or legally entitled representatives is entitled to privacy and may request confidential services. Such a request should be respected, and information obtained during such a consultation or counselling session should not be disclosed to the parents or legally entitled representatives except with the consent of the child, or in circumstances where adult confidentiality can be breached. In addition, where the attending physician has strong reason to conclude that, despite unaccompanied attendance, the child is not competent to make an informed decision about treatment, or that without parental guidance or involvement the child's health would be put in grave and irreversible danger, then in exceptional circumstances, the physician may disclose to the parents or legally entitled representatives confidential information gained during an unaccompanied attendance. However, the physician should first discuss with the child her/his reasons for doing so and attempt to persuade the child to agree to this action.

Admission to hospital

19. A child should be admitted to hospital only if the care he/she requires cannot be provided at home or on an outpatient basis.

20. A child admitted to hospital should be accommodated in an environment designed, furnished and equipped to suit her/his age and health status, and a child should not be admitted to adult accommodation except in special circumstances dictated only by her/his medical condition, e.g. where the child is admitted for childbirth or termination of pregnancy.

21. Every effort should be made to allow a child admitted to hospital to be accompanied by her/his parents or parent substitutes, who should be provided, where relevant, with appropriate accommodation in or near the hospital at no or minimal cost and with the opportunity to be absent from their place of work without prejudice to their continued employment.

22. Every child in hospital should be allowed as much outside contact and visiting as possible consistent with good care, without restriction as to the age of the visitor, except in circumstances where the attending physician has strong reason to believe that visiting would not be in the best interests of the child herself/himself.

23. Where a child of relevant age has been admitted to hospital her/his mother should not be denied the opportunity to breastfeed, unless there is a positive medical contraindication to such.

24. A child in hospital should be afforded every opportunity and facility appropriate to her/his age for play, recreation and the continuation of education, and to facilitate the latter the provision of specialised teachers should be encouraged or the child afforded access to appropriate distance learning programmes.

Child abuse

25. All appropriate measures must be taken to protect children from all forms of neglect or negligent treatment, physical and mental violence, coercion, maltreatment, injury or abuse, including sexual abuse. In this context attention is drawn to the provisions of the *WMA's Statement on Child Abuse and Neglect* (WMA Document 17.W).

Health education

26. Parents, and children appropriate to their age and/or development, should have access to, and full support in the application of, basic knowledge of child health and nutrition, including the advantages of breastfeeding, and of hygiene, environmental sanitation, the prevention of accidents, and sexual and reproductive health education.

Dignity of the patient

27. A child patient should be treated at all times with tact and understanding and with respect for her/his dignity and privacy.

28. Every effort should be made to prevent, or if that is not possible to minimise, pain and/or suffering, and to mitigate physical or emotional stress in the child patient.
29. The terminally ill child should be provided with appropriate palliative care and all the assistance necessary to make dying as comfortable and dignified as possible.

Religious assistance

30. Every effort should be made to ensure that a child patient has access to appropriate spiritual and moral comfort, including access to a minister of the religion of her/his own choice.

APPENDIX III

Average daily energy (kcal) from main food types by age and socio-economic group

| | Infants aged 6–9 months | | Infants aged 9–12 months | |
	ABC1	C2DE	ABC1	C2DE
Cereal and cereal products, of which:	89	103	193	201
Biscuits/ crispbreads	13	15	27	34
Cakes/buns/ puddings	17	21	41	42
Bread	21	20	49	44
Milk and milk products, of which:	157	171	318	299
Yoghurt	15	12	32	23
Cheese and cheese dishes	8	5	22	11
Egg and egg dishes	14	14	24	27
Fat spreads	10	11	27	25
Meat and meat products	26	24	46	47
Fish and fish products	5	4	12	8
Vegetables	6	7	13	14
Potatoes	11	13	22	30
Fruits and nuts	21	14	25	16
Sweets and preserves	9	10	14	24
Beverages, of which:	9	16	27	51
Fruit juice	3	3	6	7
Soft drinks	4	4	13	17

Continued. . .

| | Infants aged 6–9 months | | Infants aged 9–12 months | |
	ABC1	C2DE	ABC1	C2DE
Commercial infant foods, of which:	194	190	101	97
Foods in jars/ cans	60	71	38	45
Instant/dried foods	89	70	30	25
Rusks	23	29	13	16
Fruit juices	22	20	20	12
Infant formulas	165	201	29	77
Breast milk	80	33	19	10

(Source: Mills A, Tyler H. *Food and Nutrient Intakes of British Infants Aged 6–12 Months.* London: MAFF, HMSO, 1992)

APPENDIX IV

Socio-economic differences in foods eaten and amounts consumed

Foods	Non-manual (%)	Manual (%)	Non-manual (grams/week)	Manual (grams/week)
Biscuits	91	87	119	245
White bread	83	88	199	245
Non-diet soft drinks	83	87	1999	2153
Whole milk	83	83	1841	1909
Savoury snacks, e.g. crisps	77	79	77	91
Boiled, mashed and jacket potatoes	75	79	203	203
Chocolate	74	74	91	109
Potato chips	63	77	176	217
Cheese	64	54	69	67
Sweets, not chocolate	54	62	103	125
Sugar	48	59	24	40
Sausages	50	56	115	121
Chicken and turkey dishes	56	48	99	79
Pasta	56	47	246	250
Apples and pears	54	46	229	207
Baked beans	48	51	173	167
Diet drinks	52	46	1633	1713
Beef and veal dishes	47	46	183	183
Eggs	47	45	129	124
Bananas	53	40	239	228
Ice cream	47	40	127	147
Bacon and ham	44	37	58	54
Yoghurt	43	37	361	350
Leafy green vegetables	37	34	53	54
Coated or fried fish	40	37	115	116
Roast or other potatoes	34	39	72	72
Tea	29	44	559	767
Fruit juice	48	26	768	657

Continued. . .

Foods	Non-manual (%)	Manual (%)	Non-manual (grams/week)	Manual (grams/week)
Polyunsaturated margarine	41	32	35	34
Butter	34	25	25	30
Wholemeal bread	38	19	165	155
Fromage frais	32	21	227	207
Citrus fruit	31	22	188	206
Rice	23	15	173	207
Raw tomatoes	21	15	83	76
Oily fish	20	12	64	78
Pizza	14	14	164	148
Fish, not coated/ fried	13	7	112	108
Raw carrots	13	7	59	64
Canned fruit	9	7	130	147
Coffee	5	9	377	715
Mineral water	6	2	742	454
Skimmed milk	5	4	620	735
Semi-skimmed milk	33	31	1347	1086

(Source: Gregory J, Collins D, Davies P, *et al. National Diet and Nutrition Survey: children aged 1 ½ to 4 ½ years.* Ministry of Agriculture and Fisheries and Food and Department of Health. London: HMSO, 1995. © Crown Copyright material is reproduced with the permission of the Controller of Her Majesty's Stationery Office)

APPENDIX V

Excess disease rates in lower socio-economic classes and their relation to diet

Excess disease	Risk factors	Dietary contributors
Anaemia of pregnancy	Low iron, folate status	Low intake of vegetables and fruit; low intake of meat; physical inactivity
Premature delivery	Low folate; lack of n-3 fatty acids	Low intake of vegetables, fruit, and appropriate oils and fish
Low birthweight or disproportion	Adolescent pregnancy; lower folate; lack of n-3 fatty acids; low weight gain in pregnancy; smoking	Low intake of vegetables, fruit and possibly *trans* fatty acids
Anaemia in children and adults	Iron, folate, vitamins C and B_{12} deficiency	Possibly premature use of cows' milk; low intake of vegetables and fruit; low intake of meat; diet low in nutrients, with low intake linked to physical inactivity
Dental disease	Low fluoride content of drinking water	Sweet snacks and drinks between meals
Insulin dependent diabetes mellitus	Viral infections	Low breastfeeding rates
Obesity	Poor recreational facilities; intensive traffic; excessive television viewing	Physical inactivity; energy dense (high fat) diets
Hypertension	Processed foods; low birthweight	Salty, energy dense foods with high sodium and low potassium, magnesium, and calcium content; low intake of fruit and vegetables; inactivity

Continued. . .

Lipid abnormalities	Risk factors	Dietary contributors
High cholesterol	Excess weight gain	Excess dairy fats and some (hydrogenated) vegetable oils
Low high-density lipoprotein or high triglycerides	Excess weight gain	Physical inactivity; energy dense diets; low intake of fish
Non-insulin dependent diabetes	Excess weight gain	Physical inactivity; energy dense diets
Coronary artery disease	Hypertension; lipid abnormalities; smoking; low folate and antioxidants	Salty, energy dense foods with high sodium and low potassium, magnesium, and calcium; alcohol; poor intake of vegetables, fruit, and fish; low activity
Peripheral vascular disease	Smoking; low folate; lipid abnormalities	Poor intake of vegetables and fruit and possibly fish
Cerebrovascular disease	Hypertension; low folate; high cholesterol	Salty, energy dense foods high in sodium and low in magnesium, calcium, potassium; alcohol; low vegetable and fruit intake
Cancers: lung, stomach, oropharyngeal, oesophagus	Smoking with excess alcohol intake	Low intake of fruit and vegetables
Cataracts		Low intake of fruit and vegetables

(Source: James WP, Nelson M, Ralph A, *et al.* Socio economic determinants of health. The contribution of nutrition to inequalities in health. *British Medical Journal* 1997;**314**:1545–9. Reproduced with permission from the BMJ Publishing Group)

Index

Page numbers in *italics* refer to tables; those in **bold** refer to figures.

205